The Albert Plevier Trilogy
A True Love Story

Book I
Beyond the Eight-Foot World
A Chemical Plant Accident and the Journey of Pursuit

By Jayne Kelly

Jayne Kelly

Beyond the Eight-Foot World

By, Jayne Kelly

Jayne Kelly

For Al, Elaine, their Family, and Dave, because a promise made, is a promise kept, even if it takes nineteen years.

This book is additionally dedicated to the memory of the police officer who saved Al's life. Rest in peace, God Bless You.

Jayne Kelly

Table of Contents

Jayne Kelly

Introduction

$\mathscr{T}$he crisp wind traveled down from a crystal blue sky between the tall, stark buildings that sheltered High Street in Newark, New Jersey. Business people, college students, and others, clasped their coats trying to fight off hints of the impending winter from autumn's warning. Bits of trash escaped the confines of metal cans to toss and skip along the street and sidewalks. One carefree Newark School of Engineering college student braved the chill and let his coat flap open as he walked with two books clutched in one hand. He paused along his route to class for his daily ritual at the newsstand in front of the chemical engineering building and noticed the attendant was distracted.

"I'll take one Ledger." The college student, Albert Plevier, smirked as the man ritualistically ignored him. "Anything new in the world today?" Al reached into his pocket for a dime with his free hand, gave it to the attendant, and glanced at the newspaper the attendant extended. "I stopped here on my way to class to see if I *won* the draft lottery." Al fished back into his pocket for a pen and jotted down a memo across the front of the newspaper he tried to balance on his two books. His hands moved stiffly as he wrote creating an illegible script.

The newsstand attendant frowned in Al's direction. "You just better hope you don't win that lottery, Boy. That ain't no joke over there. You can't defend yourself with that diploma the school

(I)

is gonna give ya." The man snorted at Al's stack of books.

The usual humor Al used as a defense mechanism faded as he remembered the failed interview with the Air Force Academy at the end of his high school senior year. "Air Force wouldn't take me voluntarily last year." He looked distractedly up at the sky. "I'm the last male in my family in the entire country, if you can believe that."

The attendant's face softened as he seemed to suddenly stare at Al. "You got a lot to thank the Sullivan brothers for."

Al looked into the face of the disgruntled attendant. "I guess, but I want to do my part. The lottery is my ticket in. If my number comes up, I'm going. I got buddies already over there, but it'll be a while for me." Al paused for affect. "I'm number 351 out of 365." From the corner of his eye, something happening ahead on High Street caught Al's attention. He turned away from the newsstand attendant. "What's that guy doing up there?" The newspaper stand attendant never answered Al.

Crossing on High Street, along Al's route of travel, was a man out of control. He was yelling and waving a cane. People crossing High Street at the same time scattered as the man came near them. Some stared pitifully at the poor soul while others made rude comments and laughed.

That guy's gonna hurt somebody, Al thought and began to walk toward the out of control man. The man had finished crossing the busy street and narrowly avoided other pedestrians. *Poor bastard doesn't even realize how he looks to the rest of us. He must be scared or crazy or something.* Al furrowed his brow with concern, felt his forehead sting, and then the pounding of a headache began behind his eyes.

The man with the cane and Al now shared the same sidewalk. As they grew closer to each other, it was apparent the man with the cane was blind. His eyes were completely white and he appeared disheveled, but clean.

Al's headache subsided as he concentrated on the man who was now right in front of him. "Boss, do you need help?" Al didn't think the man heard him and spoke louder. "Hey, Buddy. Do you

(II)

need help?"

The head of the blind man snapped up, dislodging his chin from his chest. "Leave me be!" He jumped back and yelled nervously, "Leave me be!" His face wore the mask of a frightened soul as he shook, trying to protect himself from the unknown.

Al did not move. "Relax, Man. I'm trying to help." Al's attempt to assist the blind man was cut short by the quick jerking motion of the cane upward and toward his face. He moved back just in time and felt a cold chill as the cane passed by his face, leaving his cheek hot and burning.

Al started to back away. *Doesn't that guy know what a sideshow he's creating?*

Al stopped short one last time and called to the blind man. "Hold up. Are you okay with the direction you're going?"

"What?" The blind man momentarily calmed himself.

Al took a tentative step directly in front of the man. "I said, do you know where you are going?"

The blind man took a step backward, stumbling slightly, continued his retreat, and spoke levelly. "Stand away. I'm fine."

You're fine all right. Al thought sarcastically.

Al shook his head. "I'll see you around." Still unable to shut off his concern for the stranger, Al watched as the fading figure continued to walk erratically down High Street. The figure was becoming blurred and distorted until the blind man disappeared completely.

Looking down at his feet, Al became confused. Where were his shoes? His feet were cold. The overwhelming smell of burnt hamburger assaulted his senses. A pain shot through his head as he jolted out of the dream memory from his college days and into the reality of his bed in the Intensive Care Unit of Overlook Hospital in Summit, NJ where he lay prostrate. Everything was dark, but he knew he was awake because the pain was much too real. He heard himself scream and did not stop until more pain medication took effect.

(III)

Jayne Kelly

Chapter I: Precipice

*A*lbert Plevier, a chemical engineer and production manager for A&K Chemical Production and Supply Company of Berkeley Heights, New Jersey, paused at the water cooler on his way to the employee locker room at the end of the workday. He pulled at the collar of his shirt, anxious to change out of his sweaty work uniform. The temperature inside the warehouse production area where he spent seventy-five percent of his time climbed throughout the day in spite of the equipment for air temperature control.

Al stared at the posted green company notices above the water cooler as he grabbed a triangular paper cup from the dispenser that hung on the cooler's right side. Flipping the lever to release the water into the thin, white, paper receptacle, he felt the coolness against his fingers and quickly raised it to his lips.

He scanned the notices, drank the water, and ran an internal dialogue. *Why are all these notices green? They're usually white.* Al had grown accustomed to the constant stream of memos that flowed across his desk. *I must have missed something in my interoffice mail this morning. These are probably more OSHA memos.*

The background noise of the plant emanated from the two, open double doors on his left and reminded him that employees were still inside the production area. He continued to glance over the titles and saw today, October 1, 1974, stamped in red across the top of each paper.

Draining the paper cup of its contents he went through the mental checklist necessitated by the hour of the day. *I've seen all these notices. Maybe the office ran out of white paper. I did my final inventory check at four o'clock. All orders for today are filled and the last batch should be draining into the storage tank for pick up. I prepared tomorrow's production list. I'll be out of here before five.*

Al accepted that his title of Production Manager meant being on call twenty-four hours a day, seven days a week, but he was glad to finish each regular shift and go home for dinner with his wife Elaine and their fourteen-month-old son, Albert Junior. Changing out of his uniform was simple and quick. There were no safety gloves, goggles or helmets in the inventory available for employees. The ride home was normally an hour drive, but in his black MG at the end of a workday, he usually completed the daily commute in nearly half the time.

He reached one more time to refill the paper triangle cup letting the water saturate through the paper and dampen his fingers. While the cup began to disintegrate the sound of a motor resonated in the plant.

Still holding the cup, he tilted his head and listened intently. *What was that?* The sound had died out as quickly as it started and then sputtered to life again. *That sounds like a lawnmower.* He shook his head and continued his internal monologue. *Ain't nobody cutting grass at four-thirty in the afternoon around here.* He discerned the gas-powered-sound from the continuous hum of the plant machinery. *That sound is coming from inside the production area.* The gas motor died out.

With the saturated cup still in his hand, he turned his body left to face the propped open double doors that led to the production area. As Al listened for the motor, two loud men spoke just inside the locker room doorway in the opposite direction from where he knew the motor was located.

"Going to the baseball field?" The first voice asked.

"What do you think after being in that sweatbox for eight hours? The first day of October and it feels like summer." The two men continued to make sounds indicative of the end of a workday in a locker room.

Al considered the conversation of the two men. *Man, those two have the right idea. That sounds good. I'll jump in the MG, put the top down and run it up to ninety. What a day for it.*

The roar of the motor resonated into the corridor where Al stood and brought his thoughts back to the responsibilities of his position. *That is definitely coming from the production area. What the hell is going on in there? That's definitely not a forklift motor.*

Al heard the door of the locker room open and the footfalls of the two men who discussed the baseball game move quickly away from him toward the north exit of the plant. Confusion and then frustration over his delayed departure from the plant, combined with the knowledge that all orders were filled except the last one that was gravity draining, began to fester. He tossed the saturated cup in the garbage can at the cooler's right side, disregarding the residual water that splashed inside the plastic garbage can liner and onto the wall. Shaking his right hand to free himself of the dampness, he turned away from the water cooler and began to walk toward the production area.

His internal dialogue turned to the most likely person responsible for the interruption of his escape from the plant. *No doubt Charlie is involved in the source of that motor. What could he be doing with a gas motor in the mixing section? This guy loves to start a fresh batch of chemicals after four o'clock trying to get overtime. If that's what he's up to he'll be here 'til seven.* A working knowledge of the plant spread cold fear over his body. *That motor shouldn't have anything to do with mixing.*

Knots began to form in his stomach as Al walked through the double doors of the giant warehouse-like, production area. He was still clothed in his standard issue work uniform of an olive, green button-down shirt, matching pants, and rubber boots.

His pace quickened as his head turned from side to side scanning the area waiting for the sound of the motor. Charlie and his lack of respect for middle management stood in his mind. *That guy could have had a better deal here than anyone. I gave him a choice of using a diverter for disbursement into the drums from the storage tanks. That would have gotten him out of here by two and I would still have paid him for a full day. He wouldn't have had to start fresh batches at the end of the shift for overtime and then screw up my orders. If it was overtime pay he wanted so badly, he could make it up on the weekend shipping crew instead of inventing new ways to be here after five.*

Al had quickly traveled ten feet past the shelving for smaller containers and was now in the area of stacked pallets. These wooden pallets held four three-foot-tall drums in towers three pallets high on the right side of this main aisle. The pallets blocked the majority of Al's view of the liquid production area directly behind the pallet storage area. The motor had sputtered to life and he relied on his hearing alone to discern where it was originating from. It took a couple of seconds for him to confirm that it was coming from the right side of the main aisle, in the area where liquids, hot for both temperature and concentration, were produced. A second chill spread over him.

Voices could be heard coming from the direction of the motor. "Move it!" It was Charlie's voice ringing out clearly.

Al felt his back stiffen the minute he recognized the voice. *That's it. Whatever Charlie is up to now, it ain't worth over time.*

"Hey! Yo!" Al yelled over the motor and the continuous plant hum. He passed the first one-foot wide aisle on his right that ran between the stacked pallets of drums and could see the movement of men at the end. Believing the men to be purposely ignoring him, he made a right at the next one-foot-wide aisle and did a fast side-step shuffle to squeeze through the stacked pallets holding the storage drums.

He was coming closer to where he knew the men. *Whatever*

those guys have running, it's stationary. We use gravity to move the finished product from the mixing tanks into the storage tanks and then into the drums. The forklift trucks move the drums and there is no other need for a motor except for the truck and that's definitely not a truck. This is no good.

The motor sputtered out and then continued its brief attempts to restart, buying Al the time he desperately needed to reach the voices.

Al screamed, "Hey! Yo!," as he continued forward.

He stopped abruptly at the end of the narrow aisle. The men and motor he had searched for were five feet in front of him at the other side of a small enclosed area they had created. Al's first thought was, *"Oh my God".* The forklift truck was in front of him with a gas-powered-motorized pump sitting on the top of its forks four feet off the ground level with his upper body. The lift was positioned at an angle with the forks pointing to Al's right toward a two-story high chemical mixing tank and the rest of the truck pointing to his left. The front of the motor was pointing toward him and slightly to the left with a hose leading off the front. The final leg of the triangle, created in the small space, was a pipe vise tool that blocked any chance of escape except through the narrow aisle he had just squeezed through. The truck was positioned in a place where it was not supposed to be in order to allow the gas-powered motorized pump, that first drew Al's attention, to be between the mixing tank and the holding tank.

Al stepped into the small space as he tried to be heard over the motor that came to life again on its precarious perch. "Hey! What are you doing?" If the three men involved heard him, they ignored him. If the three men saw him, they didn't care.

One man stood on the pallet next to the pump with his back to Al. Charlie stood hunched over in the five-foot high space under the mixing tank waiting to open the quick release valve and flood the metal pipe that was utilized for gravity draining. The man on the pallet was working to start the motor and propel the hot product through the pump into a second flexible hose the size of a fire hose

(5)

that ran around the forklift truck across the floor into the waiting storage tank. A third man, who was the shift supervisor, stood off to the side of the scene watching. Al knew these men were trying to forcefully power the draining of the chemical in the mixing tank instead of using gravity. This contrived system would allow the men to empty the tank faster and mix a new batch before five. After a new batch is started, it has to be monitored and then set up to drain overnight. It was now four thirty. These men would have to stay overtime to squeeze in mixing a new batch before five. It would take only minutes to drain the current chemical mixture into the storage tank if the pump was successful. Al knew it was concentrated sodium hydroxide being transferred because, as Production Manager, he processed the orders.

Instantaneous thoughts came into Al's mind as he absorbed the imminent catastrophe. *Are these men insane? Did they rig a setup for the propulsion of twelve hundred gallons of hot chemical with a fire hose? Those clamps on the hose can't handle the pressure from the gravity release and the motor. Somebody's gonna get killed.*

The motor started and this time it did not quit. "No! No!" Al tried to be heard, waving his arms over his head trying to catch anyone's eye and he finally did.

The third man standing away from the tank snapped his head upward and then slowly backed away to a place of safety. With a horrified look on his face, the man stared back toward the motor while he crept silently into the shadows.

The motor continued to run steadily. The man who had pulled the cord to start it yelled, 'Hit it!' to Charlie who was standing underneath the mixing tank.

Charlie followed the command and opened the quick release valve, allowing hot chemicals to flood the first pipe, run into the motor, and then blast against the clamps holding the hose in place. Instantly the hose leading away from the pump broke free and hot chemicals shot out, propelled directly at Al. There was no time to move. Al stood frozen in shock, disbelief, and fear as concentrated sodium hydroxide spiraled counterclockwise toward his unprotected face and upper body. Time, in accordance with the life he was currently leading stopped. And then it hit.

"AHHHH!!" Al screamed and threw up his right arm in front of his face as the initial blast of pain from the heat and force of the liquid smashed into him.

The liquid, powered by the motor and the burning chemical, turned his feet into springs. He was blown between two metal drums and the pipe vise as the chemical concentrate kept him pinned. He was burning. He was melting. The chemical, enacting its revenge on the man responsible for diluting it, was dissolving him. The pain radiated inside his body as the chemical continued to batter the outside. Al twisted against the flood, turning and screaming as the three men at the controls scattered.

"AHHHHH! AHHHH! NOOOOOO!" Al kept up his right arm in an attempt to stop the onslaught. His screams reverberated off every wall of the warehouse and reached the front offices.

"What was that?" A secretary in the front office froze and knew she heard a man screaming. She got up from her desk to move toward the open door at the front office entrance but instead, grabbed the black phone receiver and dialed quickly. "Operator, I need the Berkeley Heights Police. This is an emergency!"

One of the three men responsible for creating the motor driven chemical accident ran into the front office screaming, just after the secretary connected to the operator and had finished her desperate request. "He's burning! He's burning!"

The operator heard the yelling and spoke calmly. "I'll send an ambulance."

The secretary froze, staring at the breathless, middle-aged man yelling at her. "Did you hear me? Get an ambulance or the cops!"

She shook herself out of the trance. "We already did."

Al, fighting to get away from the burning pain, did not know anyone was trying to help him. All he knew was that he had to save himself. He threw his body as low as he could and plastered it against the cement floor where the poison had already accumulated. The boots he was wearing were filling with burning liquid and slipped on the cement as he tried to escape.

Boxed into the small space, he began to crawl backward using the shortest route to safety. He proceeded directly through the onslaught toward the motor to get behind the force that was working to keep him pinned.

As Al fought for his life his mind screamed. *Get it off, get it off! It's going through me! I'm burning alive!*

"Ahhh, noooo!" Screaming, pushing with his unprotected hands on the slick floor his hands slipped and his internal thoughts grew into a defeated mantra. *I'm moving in place. I'm gonna die here. I'm gonna be part of the liquid. I'm melting.*

Moving backward, his mind began to drift around the pain. He realized he had reached the forklift truck the moment he no longer felt the pressure of the liquid. The mantra stopped. *I'm out!* A burst of adrenaline rose in Al and he had one thought, *Water.*

His mind started to clear as he turned to the left and reached for the truck. He found the driver's cab and pulled himself up and down the other side, dragging his battered body as he screamed nonstop. He dared to wipe the chemical from the front of his face and the skin of his forehead pulled away from his skull. Staggering toward where he knew the safety shower was, he looked through burning eyes at a world that was suddenly foggy.

Some of the skin on his hands had disintegrated, but he never saw the bits of himself he left behind as he groaned in disbelief at what had happened. He practically fell the last ten feet to the safety shower, ignoring the fog that enveloped him and grew thicker. He stepped under the eight-foot high shower head, yanked the pull chain to release the water, and felt the chain snap off. The ring still held tightly in his hands. No water, no relief.

"NOOOOOO! AHH, NOOO! ELP EEEE!" Al screamed through disintegrating lips.

Panic held its death grip on Al as he dropped the chain and

fell backward toward the slop sink he knew was on the other side of the mixing tank. He continued to scream as the bitter metallic chemical burned his tongue, destroying him now from the inside. Through the fog, Al came face-to-face with the mixing tank that stood between agony and the only relief immediately behind it. The mixing tank was five feet off the floor to facilitate the gravity fed transfer of mixed chemicals. Already hunched over, Al fell to his hands and knees screaming and crawling toward the sink. Determined to live, he moved feverishly under the tank as the fog continued to grow steadily thicker until he knew the burning in his eyes was more than just painful. He tried to raise himself up, felt space above him and moved to the sink on the right. Stumbling, he fell over into the sink and started scooping water onto his face. He became aware that people were running around him, but still not doing anything directly to help.

"Where are the cops?" a voice behind him yelled.

"I don't know, just get him to stop screaming!" came another voice.

In the middle of the confusion, a police officer arrived through the back entrance of the plant. "He's over by the sink!" One of the men directed the officer pointing toward Al who was still hanging over the sink.

Al felt his clothes being torn from his body. "Why didn't somebody get his clothes off? Get me more water!" The officer yelled desperately as he tore at Al's chemically soaked uniform and felt the chemical sear his own skin. The officer spotted a maintenance hose nearby and commanded: "Give me that hose!" The hose was brought over, the officer held it over Al's head, and the water poured down over his disappearing body. Any illusion he had that this would end as soon as more water washed over him fell away, along with the clothes at his feet. He felt his legs begin to give out beneath him as the officer's resonated in his head.

"Hang on son, hang on. The ambulance is coming. Just a little longer." The officer wasn't clear on whether the words were for himself or the damaged man in front of him.

"Awww.. ain, the ain...top the ain!" Al's lips had burned away and his words came out like a toddler.

"Hang on son, hang on. The ambulance is on the way. I hear the siren. A little longer. Hang on, son. You'll be knocked out with drugs at the hospital. Stay with me." The officer spoke as slowly as his own escalating panic would allow.

"ere?" The weakness Al felt coming over him had, momentarily, stopped the screams.

"It's in front of the plant now. Any second," the officer reassured Al. "Son, try to stand still and let the water help you. "You!" the officer turned his head to look at one of the men standing uselessly behind them. "Get over here and get these goddamn boots off him!"

The man came over and recoiled as he touched the chemical-soaked pant leg. He quickly grabbed the left boot and yanked it, almost toppling Al. As he threw the boot to the side, chemical splashed across the floor. The man started to stand to rinse his hands.

"Don't you think about it! Stay down and get the other boot off!" The officer glared at the frightened plant worker who did what the officer commanded and winced at his own pain.

The worker had gotten both Al's boots off and ran for the men's room and water.

Al barely noticed the man's presence outside his own misery. *The pain won't stop…The water isn't helping. Let me die…*

The officer kept the hose over Al's head refusing to quit his attempts to save Al's life. He switched the hose from one hand to the other as the burning chemical cut into his own skin. "You'll be in the hospital knocked out soon. Just hang on a little longer. I'm right here, and I'm not going to leave you. "Just hang on." The officer repeated the mantra and felt the promise was the only hope he could give the brutally damaged man.

"Oh, od! I aneee! I ane ee! In I eyes!" Al screamed aloud through his disintegrated lips as the fog turned to darkness.

(10)

Al could hear the arrival of the ambulance crew as the siren grew louder and then shut off. Doors opened and the sounds of a stretcher being unloaded and rushed toward him resounded in his ears, untouched by the chemical.

The attendant looked at the officer who still held the hose over Al's head. "Is he in shock?"

"No," the officer replied. "He knows what's going on. Knock him out if you can." The officer pleaded. "He needs relief."

"We can't," yelled the man in response as he and his partner pulled the stretcher next to Al.

Al nearly collapsed onto the stretcher. The ambulance attendant then got his first full view of the damage to Al. *Oh, my God. How the hell is this guy still alive? His face is melting.* "Come on sir. Ease yourself down directly behind you." The attendant guided Al.

The last thing Al wanted to do was leave the relief of the hose held above his head, but he did as he was told and hoped more water would be in the ambulance. *"Ah, no uch, ee. Ease."*

He found the stretcher, fell onto it, agony tearing through his body. Sheets clung to his wounds. The warm air so inviting earlier, now accelerated the burning.

He was loaded into the waiting ambulance twenty-five feet away. Unable to lie still, he moved and moaned as he heard the doors slam shut and felt the ambulance pull away.

"Ow ong. Ease. Ow ong." Al begged the attendant for an answer. He knew that either drugs or death awaited him at the hospital, both offering much-needed relief.

The attendant poured a container of water over Al. "Ten minutes. Hang on. The nurses will knock you out as soon as you get to the hospital." Moaning and writhing on the stretcher, Al gained a bit of control back as he listened to the attendant count the minutes to the hospital. "We're halfway there, stay with me."

Al tried to stay with the sound of the attendant's voice. "No ie, no ie." He felt desperate, like a child out of control and unable to communicate.

(11)

The attendant ran out of water and, in desperation, began to sponge it up off the floor, trying to bring about some comfort to the tortured man. "Hold on, just a few minutes more."

"Ease." Al's pleas were non-stop.

"I can see the hospital. We're pulling up to the door. They're waiting outside for us." The relief the attendant felt was both for himself and for what was left of the man on the stretcher.

Al felt himself slipping away. "Oh, od. O ore, O ore." He was growing numb.

The back doors opened and several people were around him. He was lowered quickly and rushed down a corridor. Over his screams, Al could hear the attendant speaking to someone.

"I ran out of water on the ride. He's blind. Burns are primarily on the right side of his body and face with additional damage to the feet, hands, entire chest and part of his back."

The doctor following the stretcher barked an order. "Get him in a shower!"

The quick movements intensified the pain. Al's screams now bounced off the walls of Overlook Hospital emergency room. The stretcher rounded a corner fast and then the ride came to an abrupt stop. The nurses and rescue workers brusquely pulled him up.

"Come on. Stay with us. We're in front of the shower."

The nurses sat Al on a bench inside the shower stall. There was not much left of him to cushion the drop onto the bench, and he felt the repercussion reverberate throughout his body. He heard the squeak of an old shower head begin to turn on and then water rained down over his body. Fully conscious, he finally got some of the relief he desperately needed as the water continuously ran. The last thing Al remembered was someone behind him. His screams stopped, the pain stopped and eventually so did the melting.

Chapter II: An Ordinary Day

A light breeze from the Pompton-Ramapo River carried the aroma of roasting chicken to Elaine Plevier as she cleaned the screen porch of her home. The pleasant aroma of the dinner she prepared helped her to disregard the strange feeling she had for the last half hour. It was not past her husband Al's usual time to arrive home from work, so Elaine could only attribute the nagging feeling to her pregnancy. She was in her fourth month and today the baby had made its presence known.

What a warm day it turned out to be. I should tell the girls to bring Albert outside for the last breath of the day. It won't stay like this much longer.   Elaine's sister, Ronnie, and her cousin, Cathy, were watching Albert Jr. in the living room.

It was now five-thirty. Elaine walked around the back of the house and in the open kitchen door as the phone rang.

"I'll get it," she yelled to the girls. Assuming it would be her mother, Elaine grabbed the receiver and brightly answered, "Hi, Mom."

Instead, on the other end of the phone was A&K's General Plant Manager, Anthony Milano. "Elaine, this is Mr. Milano from the plant."

"Hi." Elaine felt the nagging feeling return.

Speaking casually, Mr. Milano continued. "Elaine, there has been an accident at the plant. Nothing serious, but we did have Al taken to Overlook Hospital in Summit. You should come. I will meet you in the waiting room."

"Is it like what happened in August?" In August, chemical dust from the section of the plant where concentrated powdered chemicals were produced had irritated Al's eyes. He had to be taken to the hospital as a precaution. She found herself cradling the phone receiver under her chin and playing with her wedding band. Absent on her finger was her engagement ring whose stone she had lost two days earlier.

Mr. Milano broke into her thoughts. "No, this is a little different. Al has gotten some chemicals on his leg. This is not a problem, but I think you should go to Overlook anyway. Do you know how to get there?"

She paused slightly before answering. "Yes, I'm pretty sure I do. Are you certain this is nothing serious?" Elaine was reaching for the reassurance that her husband was safe and only inconvenienced.

Mr. Milano stuttered. "It's no big deal. Can someone drive you?" He grew impatient, wanting to end the conversation.

Elaine doubted anyone would want to spend the evening in the hospital with her. "I'll find someone. But why?"

Ignoring her question, the plant manager cut her off. "Good. I'll see you there." Mr. Milano hung up without saying goodbye.

Elaine stood with the receiver still held to her ear and decided her hormones were making her nervous. "Ronnie?"

"What's up?" Her sister looked at Elaine, anxious to leave and go out with her friends for the evening.

"That was Al's boss. I have to run to Overlook Hospital in Summit. He said Al got some chemicals spilled on his leg. Would you mind staying?" Elaine hoped she would be cooperative.

Ronnie looked over her shoulder to Cathy and the two girls

exchanged annoyed glances. Ronnie answered for both of them. "How long do you think you'll be?"

"Probably a few hours. The drive is forty-five minutes and then we might have to wait." Elaine decided that if the girls complained she would drop Albert at the neighbors. "Do you mind?"

Ronnie shrugged her shoulders and shook her head no. She pushed some loose strands of her long, blond hair behind her ear, trying to forget that she was only one hour away from what was supposed to be the end of her babysitting detail. "Don't worry about it. I hope Al is all right." She saw Elaine holding her ring finger. "Did you ever find your diamond?"

"No, and I haven't told Al. If I don't find it by the weekend, I'll tell him." She looked hard at Ronnie. "I have to run and change. Please take the dinner out of the oven in fifteen minutes and enjoy. It's herb chicken with roasted vegetables. I'll probably grab something at the hospital." Elaine deposited a kiss on Albert's head as she walked by. She heard the back door open and close but kept walking.

After she had changed she was surprised to find her mother waiting in the kitchen. "Hi, Mom. Did the girls call you?" Elaine picked up the baby and prepared to say goodbye to him.

"No, I stopped by to see if the girls were finished for the day. Ronnie said Al had an accident at work." Mrs. Hinds looked at her daughter with the baby and smiled.

"Something minor. He's at Overlook Hospital. Do you want to come along for a ride? I thought maybe we'd pick up his mom, too. You can keep each other company." Elaine walked into the living room, put the baby down on the carpet among his toys, and looked toward her mother.

"Could you send dad to pick him up instead?" Helen Hinds knew her husband would not want their pregnant daughter spending hours at a hospital emergency waiting area.

Elaine tried to reassure her mother. "I'm sure I'll have to sign papers. Dad can't do that." Elaine pictured Al impatiently waiting on a gurney in an examination room. "He'll be in a lousy mood by the time he's released."

"You're probably right." She smiled thoughtfully. "We should definitely pick up Rose. He knows his mother and I are tired after work, so he watches his manners around us."

Elaine and her mother said goodbye to the girls and Albert. Rose joined them on the journey to the hospital and the three women passed the time discussing plans for the weekend.

"It will be nice to have a family dinner on Sunday," said Elaine. "It might be one of the last ones at this house now that we have signed the contract for the Rainbow Lake house.

Mrs. Hinds gave Elaine a resigned look. "Your father's going to miss spending time by the river at the old house."

Rose Plevier gazed out the window at the changing scenery. "The house was an awful wreck when Al bought it, but what a beautiful job he has done."

"Yes, he certainly has," Elaine answered trying not to sound sarcastic as she thought of the work she and Al had completed together

Mrs. Hinds, feeling the tense tone in her daughter's voice, tried to lighten the mood. "Rose and I could both come up to help you with the packing this weekend. You don't want to do too much with the new baby coming."

Rose smiled at her friend and in-law. "I think that would be fun. We could help with the cooking and with Albert."

A sense of contributing and the thought of the family being together this weekend brought a feeling of peace to Rose. The home her son and daughter-in-law had purchased was becoming the central anchor for their extended families. Located on the river, originally in a rural area, the house had been a lodge that served as a great escape for many well-known individuals, including Babe Ruth. Al's love of baseball made this house special to him and it was difficult to consider selling it. Both Al and Elaine struggled with the decision to sell the house but realized together that the Lake Road house they now lived in was a starter home and their young family was quickly outgrowing it.

The plans the three formulated for the weekend ahead made

the drive to Overlook Hospital easy and even enjoyable. Elaine had begun to forget her uneasy feelings until she parked the car around six-thirty that evening.

Already in the lobby, Mr. Milano greeted the women tersely. "The waiting area is over here." He nodded in the direction of a bland room with a few seated people to the right of the group

Walking alongside him, Elaine stopped short and looked up into his eyes inquiring, "Has Al come out?"

Gazing past Elaine, toward nothing in particular, he replied, "No, not yet."

Not yet? For a simple mishap? Why is Mr. Milano here?

Elaine immediately walked toward the nurses' station and did not notice Mr. Milano had dropped away from her. "Excuse me. I'm here for Albert Plevier. His boss said that he hasn't come out yet and I was wondering..."

The nurse interrupted Elaine. "Someone will be with you as soon as we know something." The nurse began to turn back to the doorway behind her.

"Know something?" Elaine was left to stare at the empty space left by the nurse's departure. She turned to her mother and mother-in-law who had found seats in the waiting area.

"What did the nurse say, Hon?" Helen Hinds asked nervously.

Not wanting to worry the two women, Elaine spoke as nonchalantly as she could. "Oh, you know hospitals, Mom. He's lost somewhere in the back among the paperwork." She found a seat next to her mother and the three began waiting.

"Mom, I realized that I didn't have dinner. Would you run to the cafeteria for me?"

"Sure. Do you want something specific or will anything do?" Mrs. Hinds fished inside her purse for her wallet.

"Try to make it something healthy," Elaine said as she rubbed her stomach, thinking of the new pregnancy that was beginning to show. "But, at this point, anything will do." She not only needed food, she needed the opportunity to approach a nurse without the attention of either woman. "Why don't you keep Mom company, Rose?"

When the two women were out of sight, Elaine walked to the nurse's desk and approached a different nurse. "Excuse me please, I'm here for Albert Plevier. No one has told me anything. I don't even know what exactly happened."

The nurse gave Elaine a strange look before she replied. "As soon as the doctors can, one will come out and talk with you about Mr. Plevier."

Doctors? He needs more than one? Something's wrong. Out of the corner of her eye, Elaine was sure she saw Mr. Milano wince as he stood across the emergency room from her. She started to walk toward him and he quickly walked away, leaving Elaine to stare into empty space.

Mrs. Hinds and Rose arrived back from the cafeteria with an assortment of fruit and two wrapped sandwiches. "I hope this will do, dear," Rose offered apologetically.

"That's fine. The doctor still has not come out, and the nurse won't tell me anything. I'm not sure what to make of all this." Elaine no longer tried to hide her apprehension.

Mrs. Hinds offered the simplest explanation. "Honey," she paused briefly for emphasis, "I'm sure the delay is procedural nonsense. Al is probably screaming to come home."

A sense of foreboding enveloped the three women as an anonymous voice came over the intercom system. "Would Mrs. Plevier please come to the lobby desk for a phone call."

Elaine's felt herself become nauseous. "Mom, would you please go see if the call is from Ronnie and Cathy? I don't want to leave the ER in case the doctor comes out."

Mrs. Hinds reached out and patted her daughter's arm. "Sure, Hon."

A few moments later Mrs. Hinds returned to find Elaine and Al's mother silent and still sitting in the same chairs. As she walked toward them she saw Mr. Milano, who had come from another direction leaning against a wall. From where the other two women sat he was out of sight. Her eyes met his and she stared at him, watching as the color drained from his face. Her gait slowed as she approached her daughter.

Elaine looked up from the magazine she was blankly staring at and felt her mother come close to her. "Mom? What is it?"

Fighting back the knot that had formed in her throat, she spoke. "Elaine that was Fenna, not the girls." She struggled to find words.

Elaine grew stiff both from the look on her mother's face and the new knowledge that Al's sister had called. Thoughts raced through her mind. *Why would Fenna call? How did she know about this? Who told her? She has her own family to worry about.* "Mom, what *is* it?"

Mrs. Hinds looked at the floor and then the ceiling as she fought back tears. "Fenna called the hospital earlier after talking to the girls." Mrs. Hinds had to stop before going on. "She had called the house to talk to you about getting together this weekend. The only reason she called the hospital was because it was the second time in six months that something happened at that plant."

Elaine mistakenly thought the anger in her mother's voice was directed at the circumstances, instead of at the man she had just faced down in the corridor. Elaine and Rose gripped hands.

Elaine rose from her chair still holding her mother-in-law's hand. "Mom, what did she say?"

Looking into her daughter's eyes Helen Hinds continued. "A nurse told her that he was being operated on. Fenna called us to see if we knew anything else." The emptiness in the woman's voice hung before Elaine like an ominous black cloud.

Mr. Milano moved from the wall he had leaned against toward the three women still offering nothing. Elaine managed to find her voice, looked up, stared directly at him and spoke loudly. "What is going on?"

Mr. Milano opened his mouth to respond, looked down at his shoes, and then mumbled to no one in particular, "Al's being taken care of," and walked away.

Elaine, Helen Hinds, and Rose Plevier were left to stare at

Mr. Milano's receding back until he turned left at the first corridor available to him. The nagging feeling Elaine had for the last couple of hours was now replaced with a coldness that spread from her chest to every point in her body. She started to walk toward the nurse's station as a man in a white lab coat approached her from the triage entrance double doors.

"Is Mrs. Plevier here?" The man in the white lab coat looked between Elaine, Mrs. Hinds, Al's mother, and two other women walking through the waiting area with coffee.

"Yes," Elaine replied flatly, staring at the doctor.

The man, who had looked rushed upon entering the waiting area paused as he looked at the young woman before him. "Mrs. Plevier, Albert is still in surgery and that is all we know." Elaine did not respond and he continued. "The doctors who are taking care of him will be out soon. I'm sorry but I have a car accident coming in." The man turned and quickly retreated into the triage area.

"Mom," was all Elaine could manage as she turned toward her mother for support.

Rose Plevier and Mrs. Hinds guided Elaine back to a chair as the two women with the coffee sat down across from them, engrossed in their own drama and tragedy. For the next several hours, people came and went into the waiting area and adjoining corridor, but the women hardly noticed.

The uncomfortable orange, plastic seat Elaine sat in had become warm but unforgiving. She had stopped shifting her expanding body from side to side in a vain attempt to alleviate the building aches. Around her, the beige walls started to close in. She looked up to notice stains on the ceiling, but she soon became too dizzy to concentrate on them. Her eyes found a place to rest and she tried to focus on the black swirls that made up the design on the linoleum floor. The conversation between the women was kept to a minimum.

Outside of the waiting room void, a loud, male voice called from the open triage door. "Mrs. Plevier?" A weary looking man wearing a physician's jacket stood outside the triage double doors.

Elaine rose stiffly, moving toward the doctor she hoped would give her answers. She was followed closely by the two mothers. "I'm Elaine Plevier, Albert's wife."

With no hand extended the doctor introduced himself. "I'm Dr. Westmont, the physician your husband's care was placed in." Dr. Westmont looked directly into Elaine's eyes and saw little reaction. "The chemical has left Albert blind. He has burns over sixty percent of his body, primarily on the right side, back, face and part of the left side of his torso. The second-degree burn damage is on his legs and feet. There is third-degree damage on the remaining affected areas. These are caustic burns from a base chemical. If it was an acid burn it would have burned the skin, but since it was a base, the body started to absorb the chemical and tried to destroy the affected areas. I can give you no definitive answers as to the outcome of his survival." Dr. Westmont paused before continuing glancing at the two women who stood on either side of Elaine with their hands over their mouths and tears in their eyes. "You and your family should be prepared for the possibility that Albert may not survive the night."

Elaine stared at Dr. Westmont without responding. She heard the sharp intakes of breath on either side of her.

"Mrs. Plevier?" Dr. Westmont, emotionless, tried to hold the women in the moment, however brutal that moment was for them.

"May not survive the night?" Elaine stood in shock before the doctor, unable to scream, cry, or move.

The antiseptic composure of Dr. Westmont erased itself. He stared at her blank expression quizzically, but with horror. "No one explained to you what happened to your husband at work today?" Elaine and the two women began to shake their heads slowly and Dr. Westmont drew in a quick breath before he continued. "I'm so sorry. I assumed you were told all about the accident that had taken place. The plant manager has been here since the ambulance arrived."

Anger and began to grow inside Elaine. "Please, tell me what happened to my husband." Her voice grew loud enough to draw the attention of other people in the waiting area as she stared directly into the eyes of Dr. Westmont not moving from her place.

Dr. Westmont looked at each of the women before continuing. "Albert has been sprayed with a highly, concentrated form of sodium hydroxide. As I explained this is a base and not an acid. The body absorbed it in the areas of destruction and started to dissolve the tissue. He is in intensive care and should not have visitors until we can reassess his progress. If we feel that he is not improving tonight," Dr. Westmont stopped short and looked briefly at the floor. "We will call you at home so that you can be at his side. You cannot help him by waiting here. It would be better for you and your family if you went home." Dr. Westmont tried to emphasize the word 'home' to the women in front of him.

Dazed, confused, and still trying to grasp the alternative reality she had been thrown into, Elaine felt a hand placed on her shoulder. She looked over her shoulder at her mother's tear stained face, and then looked toward the doors that led to the triage area. "How did this happen?" She directed the question to the world in general.

He looked at Elaine with compassion that he controlled as he maintained his professional demeanor. "I don't know the exact events that led to the accident. Our concern tonight is keeping him alive. We are making every effort to salvage his eyes for the future possibility of regaining his sight, but as I have said, our immediate concern is keeping him alive." After receiving no response from the three women, Dr. Westmont continued. "It would be best if you went home and tried to get some rest. You can call the desk throughout the night to check on his condition. If you stay at the hospital, I will not allow you to see Albert unless his condition worsens."

Elaine's mom spoke to her in a voice that was close to a whisper. "We need to get you home. You have to think of the baby." The older woman placed her hand on her daughter's arm.

Elaine looked at her mother, breathed deeply, and lifted her eyes to meet the doctors. "No. I can't leave Al here alone." She felt her voice break. "He can't be here all alone." Elaine bowed her head to hide the tears that were now falling freely. Dr. Westmont was silent and let his gaze travel between the two older women. Elaine broke the silence. "I can't leave here."

Mrs. Hinds tried to lessen the shock her daughter had just experienced. "You need to lie down. You can't do that here." She managed to turn Elaine around and look into her broken face. "You can't stay here all night. You just can't do it."

Panic replaced the numbness that had gripped Elaine. "What if something happens? Let me sit in the waiting room."

Dr. Westmont broke in. "He is holding his own for now. He is in no pain. You will be allowed to see him tomorrow. If you don't go home and rest, you won't be able to understand everything that will be explained to you tomorrow as he progresses." *If he progresses.* The doctor could not be certain.

Silence enveloped the group as Elaine gathered herself and then looked back up at Dr. Westmont with resignation in her eyes. "I'll be calling all night. We'll be back first thing in the morning. If he regains consciousness, you tell him we'll be in to see him soon." *He needs me. Why do they want me to leave?*

Dr. Westmont thought, *I will not let this man regain consciousness tonight. He has been through enough torture for one day.* He looked down into Elaine's eyes. "I promise to have you called if he wakes up."

The three women composed themselves before Mrs. Hinds broke the silence. "Please, Elaine. Let's get you home. All she could think of was to get her daughter to a place where she could take care of her. The waiting area was nothing more than purgatory. There was another baby at home waiting for his mother. "Please, Elaine." She began to pull gently on her daughter's arm.

Helen's thoughts were so focused on her own daughter that she struggled to focus on the despair her friend and in-law, Rose Plevier, must be feeling. She watched Rose's blank stare fall to the linoleum floor in front of her. Helen knew, in that moment, that she had to be the strength to guide Elaine and Rose out of the black, sterile hole they had been thrown into.

"We can stop at phone booths on the way home if you would like to call the hospital. I'll drive." She began to lead Elaine and Rose out of the waiting area.

Rose struggled to lift her weighted eyes and over her shoulder saw Mr. Milano come, seemingly out of the shadows, to speak to Dr. Westmont.

Elaine did not see Mr. Milano and he never looked at the three women who walked out of the waiting room and through the doors leading to the parking area. She stepped out of the hospital and felt the crisp, fall night air dry the tears on her cheeks and bring her out of the shock she had just experienced.

She stopped and looked back at the hospital building.
Al, oh God, how did this happen? This isn't real. I don't want to leave you. Please God, help him. Help him to hold on. Don't leave me, Al. Just live.

Finding the car was not difficult at this time of the evening. The three women climbed inside the station wagon without asking where each would sit. Mrs. Hinds got behind the wheel and the drive back to Wayne was silent except for the occasional quiet sob or sniffling. Mrs. Hinds dropped Rose at her daughter Fenna's home. Fenna stood waiting at the door, her body a silhouette against the inside light. Rose Plevier walked up the steps, met her daughter, and both women visibly shook.

Mrs. Hinds pulled the car away without speaking, knowing her friend Rose was now being taken care of. She was eager to get her daughter home to rest and sort through the recent shock in a more comforting environment. The car pulled into the circular driveway of Al and Elaine's home and Helen could see Ronnie, Cathy, and Mr. Hinds get out of their chairs.

Elaine opened the car door. Her arms and legs felt strangely heavy as she leaned against the tan vinyl door until the metal weight gave way. She wondered, offhandedly, if her legs would support her before she climbed out of the car and shut the door behind her. Sluggishly she found her way to the kitchen door. Brief words of comfort, hugs, and tears blocked her entrance until the women walked together and then sat down at the kitchen breakfast bar.

Cathy spoke first. "Elaine, I called my mom while you were at the hospital. She knows one of the nurses at Overlook." She absorbed the exhausted, pale look on Elaine's face. "I wanted to get you any extra information that we could."

"What did Aunt Catherine tell you," was all Elaine could manage.

Mr. Hinds came over, hugged his daughter wordlessly and then sat hard at the counter staring into space.

Cathy tried to repeat everything verbatim her mother had told her. "There is intense damage done to his body and eyes. He has been burned on approximately sixty percent of his body. Thirty to forty percent of his body mass has been melted away. The doctors are not sure at this point if he will ever see but there is an effort to try to salvage the eyes. His face may be unrecognizable." Cathy stopped short, unsure if she said too much.

Elaine looked up at Cathy between strands of hair that had fallen in her face. "Finish, please."

Cathy looked at her hands and then over to Helen. "Elaine, his face is badly burned. I'm sorry. I don't know what he will look like when you see him tomorrow."

Elaine looked past Cathy and into the living room behind her. "The pain he is in must be horrible. I hope the doctors have him heavily sedated. I don't want him to feel any more pain than he has to."

Silence descended on the room. Elaine pushed away from the breakfast bar, got up from her chair, and walked across the living room to the hallway without looking back or speaking. She hesitated at the closed nursery door and took a deep breath to calm her nerves. Quietly and slowly she opened the door and approached the crib to look down upon her fourteen-month-old son Albert. The powder fresh smell of the baby was a comforting stark contradiction to the hospital smell she had just left behind. She felt the polarity of life and death as she reached down and touched the back of her sleeping baby. New tears fell from her eyes, falling from her cheeks as she wondered about what the future might hold for the two of them.

I can't believe fate would be so cruel to allow Al's children to lose their father. Al barely remembers his dad. He wants to be the father to his children that his own father never had the chance to be. God, please, don't take that away from him, away from these children, or from me. I love him so much. I will accept whatever Al's condition will be. Get him through tonight.

Chapter III: Rude Awakening

*R*ising before the sun after sleeping intermittently through the long night, Elaine reached across the queen-sized bed for the husband who was not there. She had called the hospital every hour and heard the same consistent report: "There is no change Mrs. Plevier. He is holding his own."

Fresh tears fell down her cheeks as she focused on the daisy print comforter she had purchased in the spring. She thought about her husband's reaction to the purchase: "I feel like I'm sleeping in a garden. I'm not an old lady. Get rid of this thing."

The air around Elaine was thick with the weight of the previous night and what might lie ahead today. Across the hall, she heard her son stirring and found the strength to climb out of bed. She walked toward the half-closed nursery room door and pushed it open. Little Al immediately rolled to his knees and pulled himself to a standing position inside the crib.

"Mama," he chanted as he held out his arms.

I'm here, little man. How did you sleep?" Elaine scooped the little boy out of his crib. The warmth of her baby and his arms around her neck brought immediate comfort. Albert pointed to the doorway. "Not yet. Let's get you changed and then we'll go see who is here."

Elaine had known someone from her family was still in the house by the movement she heard beyond the walls of the master bedroom. She had only guessed that someone would stay with the baby if, God forbid, Al had taken a turn for the worse during the night and she needed to drive to Overlook.

She changed, dressed, and carried the baby to the living room. Immediately he squirmed to be put down and then ran across the room to his Grandpa. "Papa," he said excitedly.

"Come here, big guy. How ya doing?" Mr. Hinds picked Little Albert up and gave him a hug. He then looked over at his pale, exhausted daughter. "Honey, come sit. Have a little coffee."

Elaine gave a grateful half smile to her Dad and approached the counter. "Thanks, Dad. No coffee for me. The new baby." She patted her stomach, sat down at the breakfast bar, and rubbed her eyes with the palms of her hands.

"I'll go with you today." Mr. Hinds looked at his daughter through the tired eyes of a father who had been awake all night.

Elaine was both anxious to see Al and dreaded it at the same time. How could she watch her husband suffer? The fear was overtaken by the thought that she had to be near him. Since High School, she had never let more than two days pass without at least talking to him, even after a brief break up.

Elaine's mother came into the living room and placed her hand on her shoulder. "How about something to eat?"

"I don't know that I can keep anything down." Elaine still held her hand on her stomach and thought about her unborn child. "I know I should, but maybe toast with butter will work. I'll have it after I take my shower."

Elaine picked up the receiver of the yellow kitchen phone next to the counter and dialed the hospital number. Mr. and Mrs. Hinds looked at each other and then both focused on Albert.

Elaine heard a new voice answer. "ICU."

"This is Mrs. Plevier. I am calling to check on my husband." As with all the previous calls, she felt a twisting nauseating sensation in her stomach as she waited for a response.

"He's holding his own." The nurse responded with a coldness Elaine did not expect.

"My family and I will be at the hospital within the next two hours. I will be driving so you will not be able to reach me." Elaine did not want to hang up the phone and leave Al in the hands of this impersonal, unemotional woman.

"Thank you." The nurse hung up before Elaine could continue the conversation.

She stared at the receiver in her hand before hanging it back on the wall. "I need to hurry and get to the hospital. Dad, are you ready?"

"Ronnie is already on her way over to watch Little Albert. Your mom and I will drive with you. Fenna and Al's mom will meet us there." Mr. Hinds spoke to Elaine as he watched her wordlessly push away from the counter and cross the living room toward the master bedroom and bath. "Elaine, he made it through the night. He's going to survive." Elaine did not respond.

She showered, dressed and came back out of the master bedroom with the stride of a robot. "Dad?"

Mrs. Hinds was in the kitchen with Ronnie. "Dad is outside warming up the car." Elaine watched Ronnie feeding and talking to Albert. "Are you ready, Hon?" Ronnie lifted Albert out of his high chair and carried the little boy toward his mother.

Elaine kissed him quickly. "I'm ready. Ronnie, please make sure he eats today. We'll call as soon as we know anything."

Albert, oblivious to the events of the last twenty-four hours, gripped his stuffed snoopy with one arm and his Aunt Ronnie with the other. "Elaine, I'll take care of everything. I called work early this morning and told them I had a family emergency."

Elaine picked up her purse and walked out the door without saying goodbye. She got into the back seat of the station wagon, grateful to relinquish driving to her dad.

(29)

Numbness began to creep into Elaine's body and she spoke aloud to try and break the spell. "I told Ronnie we would check in every couple of hours."

Mr. Hinds looked over his shoulder. "I'm sure she'll take good care of the baby."

Elaine nodded in acknowledgment and then stared out the window looking at the edge of the circular driveway. Thoughts of her sister taking over her duties for the day climbed into her consciousness. Elaine had always been the strong, smart, and responsible one who made all the right choices. Al had always described the difference between the two women as cotton balls and seashells. Elaine was the cotton balls. Now she had to trust her sister to take care of a piece of her heart while she traveled to the hospital to make sure the doctors were taking care of another.

She noticed nothing as the roadway and its accompanying scenery rushed past the windows of the car. Upon their arrival at the hospital, Mr. Hinds dropped the two women at the front entrance before proceeding to park the station wagon.

Elaine and her mother walked stoically to the front desk and were met halfway by Fenna and Rose Plevier. "Mom." Elaine embraced her mother-in-law solidly, something the two women were not accustomed to doing and then all four women turned to the nurses' station.

Mrs. Hinds spoke before Elaine had a chance to gather her thoughts. "Excuse me. Could you please direct us to the ICU?"

The receptionist spoke to the women without consideration of the recent family trauma. "You aren't allowed into the ICU unit until you have proper instructions."

Mrs. Hinds drew in her breath before speaking. "We understand that. We are here to meet first with Dr. Westmont, the doctor in charge of my son-in-law's care. He was severely burned yesterday."

The young woman behind the desk flushed with embarrassment. "I'm so sorry. Please, let me find out where Dr. Westmont is." She began to dial numbers and after listening to the voice on the other end, spoke to Elaine. "The doctor was in the ICU and he is on his way down to speak with you."

Elaine found this last information comforting. "Thank you."

Mr. Hinds had returned from parking the car when he saw Dr. Westmont walk up to the group. The doctor motioned with his hand for everyone to follow him. Elaine found herself walking down a long corridor with many doors on either side. Each door had glass on the upper half.

Dr. Westmont looked over the exhausted group in front of him when they reached a tiny alcove with water fountains. "Albert survived the night and is improving slightly."

Relief swept over Elaine. "Can he have visitors?"

The intercom spoke somewhere in the hallway ahead of the group. "Dr. Westmont, you have a call waiting."

"I have to take this. Please follow me." Dr. Westmont continued a few steps ahead of them. "You will be seeing your husband in a few minutes, but we have to acquaint you with the procedures. You're as much a danger to him as the common cold right now." He reached for the phone on the upper-level counter of the nurses' station, punched in the necessary code and announced himself. "Dr. Westmont."

Elaine watched the man who held her family's future in his hands speak with the ease of a professional to the party at the other end of the phone. A sense of confidence began to develop beneath the panic and dread that consumed her.

Dr. Westmont hung up the phone and turned back to Elaine and the family members. "First we need gowns for you to wear. Only two of you will be allowed in. Please decide who."

There was no decision to be made. After hugging her mom, Elaine reached for Rose Plevier's hand, and the two women walked beside the doctor as Mr. and Mrs. Hinds and Fenna stayed back and watched the women disappear around a bend in the corridor. Dr. Westmont held the door for the two women at the dressing area entrance half way down the hall. Elaine let go of her mother-in-law's hand and felt her knees become weak.

"Please put the gowns over your clothes, tie the hat to cover all of your hair, put the mask on to cover your nose and mouth, place the booties over your shoes and lastly, please remember to put on the protective gloves." The doctor stepped back out of the room and waited by the door.

"Mom, can you get the booties on?" Elaine hurriedly dressed, hoping her mother-in-law would do the same.

"Yes, I'm doing fine." The older woman kept her gaze to the floor as she dressed. A constant thought ran through her mind repeatedly: *Little children should not lose their fathers. I watched Al cry as his heart broke at age five over the death of his father. He has to live.*

Completely dressed from head to toe in protective garments, the two women proceeded through the doorway to Dr. Westmont. "Doctor, does Al know the extent of his injuries? Did he awaken at all? Has he spoken to anyone?" Her questions were a desperate attempt for acknowledgment of a miracle.

"We are keeping him sedated as much as possible. He won't be fully conscious for at least two weeks. His body has experienced a terrible shock." Dr. Westmont finished speaking as the sound of machines beeping could be heard on the other side of a door.

The woman and the doctor stood in an outer room that was separated from an adjoining room by a glass paneled door and large glass partitions. Through the glass partition, Elaine could see a body lying on a mesh type hospital bed. The body was naked except for a sheet draped over a plastic tent. She caught her breath as she saw the face, swollen and discolored. It bore no resemblance to her husband.

For a second, she thought it was the wrong room. Denial washed over her as she stared at the shattered human being lying with tubes and oozing wounds underneath the covering.

"Mrs. Plevier?" Dr. Westmont saw the pale faces and tears in the eyes of the two women.

Elaine tore her gaze away from Al and looked down to the floor. "Let me gather myself."

(32)

A hand touched Elaine's right shoulder and she turned to look into the eyes of her mother-in-law. It would not be until years later when Elaine looked back at this, that she would marvel at how Al's mother did not crumble on the floor. Rose Plevier watched her adult child through the glass partition as he suffered near death and summoned the emotional fortitude to support her daughter-in-law. She stood with her hand on Elaine's right shoulder, offering the strength of her years and the love in her heart.

The two women were surrounded by the dry, antiseptic, empty air that accompanies hospitals. As the doctor held open the inner door to where Al lay, the smell of burnt hamburger assaulted their senses. The smell replaced the hope for life with the real possibility of death. Elaine and Rose moved together through the door holding one hand in front of the surgical masks that covered their mouths and noses. The vain attempt to block the acrid, strong, nauseating smell that was now a part of Al did not work.

The two women moved toward the bedside until Elaine felt Rose take one step back directly to Elaine's right as she kept one hand on Elaine's shoulder propelling her toward her husband's bedside. The older woman gathered all the intensity and love she had for her son and his family and gave his wife her rightful place at her husband's side.

Elaine did not immediately move to Al's bedside, afraid of the protective tent that held his body. One of the nurses moved in front of her and pulled back the sheet that hung like a tent over Al. The damage the sodium hydroxide had caused became fully visible to the two women. Elaine focused first on his feet and then slowly moved her gaze upward. As she studied his body intently, she could only imagine the pain he was in. His feet were swollen, red, bleeding and oozing where the outer layer of his skin used to be. Ugly red spots blotched and speckled his ankles, calves and left thigh, but the real damage increased as her gaze moved upward. His right thigh was a flame red that became black up his right side and over his chest where more bleeding and oozing was taking place. His torso appeared concave. Al's right arm was elevated on a table and cushioned with soft fabric she didn't recognize. The

(33)

left arm fared better and served the purpose of funneling all the liquids and medications necessary for his survival into his bloodstream. It took every bit of her strength to move her gaze above his neck. After closing her eyes briefly, she opened them.

He looks like a monster. Oh, God. His head looks like a giant black pumpkin. She quickly squeezed her eyes shut as her thoughts betrayed her. *He has no lips. Most of his hair is gone. Will he ever be the same? His eyes are covered with bandages. Will he ever see again?*

Tubes ran out of both Al's eyes underneath the bandages. A larger tube inserted into his nose looked uncomfortable and nauseating, but she was shocked to not see a tracheotomy or a tube coming from his mouth. Hope rose inside her as she realized he was, at least, breathing on his own and had not inhaled the chemical. Elaine carefully approached his bedside, aware of the bag hanging from the bed railing outside the protective tent that captured what the catheter drained. A small table next to his bed held instruments, medications and various medical necessities.

With her throat seized and dry, Elaine steeled herself silently praying that her fear did not present itself to her husband in her voice. She needed him to know she was with him as she took a step closer to his head and leaned as far as the protective tent would allow her.

"Al, I'm here." The brief acknowledgment of her presence was all she could manage before straightening to regain her composure. She knew he was heavily medicated and leaning over, fought her emotions as she let tears slide down her cheeks. "Keep fighting, Al. We'll get through this." Believing Al to be in sedated oblivion, Elaine was shocked to hear sounds coming from him.

"aine…aine….."

She put her hand to her mouth as she kept her head near his to try to understand what he struggled to say beneath lips that had disappeared.

"Lor tol ee id ill ee awight."

Startled, Elaine responded stoically. "Your mom is also by your bedside, Sweetheart. We will get through this. Everyone is helping with the baby and with me. I love you so much." Elaine straightened and stepped aside to guide her mother-in-law next to Al's bed.

Rose struggled to find her voice. "Son, I'm here and I love you. Keep fighting your way back to us. Your family needs you." Rose Plevier covered her mouth to conceal a cry that almost escaped.

"I think that is enough for now, please." Dr. Westmont spoke from the doorway. "He knows you're here, but he needs to stay sedated. We can go out into the lounge with your other relatives and discuss what is going to happen over the next four days."

Elaine kept her eyes on her husband until she was forced to turn to the doorway. It was not lost on her that Dr. Westmont had said he wanted to speak about what was going to happen in the next couple of days and not the next several weeks. Al's condition was being considered one hour to the next and each day he lived was a miracle. Dr. Westmont walked with the women to the lounge area where the family waited.

Elaine was the first to speak. "Dr. Westmont, how are we going to help him?" Tears broke through the last word she spoke.

The doctor looked down at the chart he clutched and wore the mask of a professional determined to do his job. "I feel that we may have success with the burn tissue down the road, but right now I would like to explain to you about the damage done to his eyes." He scanned the people in front of him and then turned his gaze to Elaine. "It might be helpful in the future if one person took notes on some of the directives that I lay out for you. It will be imperative that you have notes logging his medication and initial care given and that you keep a record of it to refer back to." He paused for effect. "I feel that Albert will survive this. He's young, healthy and strong. He can live a long and happy life, but the choices you make concerning his recovery will decide how that will happen." Dr. Westmont looked hard into Elaine's eyes. "This is a lifelong condition. He cannot be cured, but he can continue to recover." The last sentence spoken hung heavily in the air.

Fenna spoke up and brought to the forefront the practical questions that needed to be answered. "How long will Al remain in the hospital? How long will he remain in ICU?"

"Minimally, assuming he continues to make progress, we are talking at least two months in the hospital, depending on his recovery process. We would like to see him leave ICU within ten days, but there are a lot of variables that can affect that. His burns, however, will not be healed in that time period. The severity of the burns will require constant attention for years," Dr. Westmont looked at Elaine. "Let's talk about Albert's eyes. You need to understand what has happened and what may continue to happen. The chemical that assaulted his body, sodium hydroxide, has reacted with the cornea, the protective lens that covers the eye and acts as a window. It didn't take long during the accident for Albert's vision to cloud up and finally be compromised. We have placed experimental medicine into his eyes to pull out the chemical that remained after the water rinsed out as much as possible. I used the experimental drug because, to be quite frank, he had nothing left to lose. If we had not used it initially the sodium hydroxide would have already eaten through the cornea and destroyed the optic nerve where it connects to the retina totally destroying any future possibility of regaining vision. These are layman's terms, but I assume that if you would need or are ready for further explanation, you would feel free to ask."

"What are the chances of his sight returning?" Elaine's thoughts were not organized and the obvious question was all she could manage.

"Beyond that question lies the mystery as to what degree it would return at all." Dr. Westmont responded honestly. "The ordeal you and your family will endure is just beginning, Mrs. Plevier. We will continue to discuss the possibility of his sight returning, but let's focus on his initial recovery first."

Shocked by the condition of Al's injuries, Dr. Westmont's speculation at least gave Elaine something to work with. "Thank you for saving my husband's life." Her thoughts returned to Al.

The wounded body she left in the Intensive Care Unit was

a mass of oozing, burned tissue that did not resemble her husband. The body she saw looked like it would not survive the next few moments, let alone another day. She was terrified. The simple pattern to life that she knew, the pattern that her parents had taught her: to work hard, gain knowledge, fall in love, put everything you've learned into practice, and move ahead, no longer applied. Her little family was in survival mode.

The next words she spoke aloud were more for herself than anyone in the extended family. "I know Al will pull through this. After he regains consciousness he will need to know there is a chance for his sight to return."

The seasoned physician spoke with frank experience to Elaine and now turned to the family members gathered. "I feel I must tell you that Albert will have a tremendous need for you toward the end of his stay here and even more after he goes home." He looked over the faces that stood around him for a reaction to confirm that everyone grasped the new reality. "You have to think about conserving the family energy for that time." He stopped speaking and looked at the large aluminum clock that hung inside the waiting area. "If you stay today you will not be permitted back inside the ICU room." He continued to look hard into the faces before him. "I'll be in the hospital for most of the day. If you have questions, you can leave messages with my service, and I will return your call. Please consider going home and absorbing all of this. You can't do anything for Albert at the immediate moment." Dr. Westmont looked from one family member to the next then nodded perfunctorily and walked back through the double doors that led to the ICU unit.

Elaine, still trying to digest the events of the last twenty-four hours, lifted her eyes to meet her mother's. "I think he's trying to be professional." At least she hoped that was the case as the family members found their way to the same orange chairs Elaine had spent last evening seated in.

The exercise of scheduling their lives began to formulate in Mr. Hind's mind and he gripped his hands tightly together as he looked over at his daughter. "We all need to work through this as a team. Elaine, you can't expect to handle everything alone. What we need to do now is think about the logistics of getting you to the hospital, while having constant care for the baby."

Fenna spoke next. "Maybe it would help if mom and I came up to the hospital in the morning before her work shift. I can get the woman next door to watch my kids. Elaine can then have her mornings with Albert until one of her neighbors can watch him for an hour or two until either Ronnie or Elaine's parent's come home from work." She looked into Elaine's weary face. "Will you be able to do the drive alone every day?" Fenna tried to draw Elaine's focus back to the conversation after watching her gaze drift catatonically out the windows into the parking area.

"Yes. I'll be fine. I just wish I could be here all the time." Elaine's cheeks had lost their color.

Mrs. Hinds reached over and took her daughter's hands. "On the weekend, other family members will be able to help. You'll see Al all the time."

Rose Plevier moved her hand away from her mouth where it had been since she sat down. "He is in the hands of the best doctors in the area."

Al's mother was approaching retirement and thought the hardest years of her life were behind her. She had survived the Depression as a young girl and the death of her husband as a young bride, but the ability to survive those challenges did not give her the strength to watch her son suffer. She was completely numb.

The small group ignored the doctor's suggestion to go home and spent the rest of the day at the hospital, grasping for any small improvement in Al's condition. At six that evening the group left in two separate cars with the visitation plan for the next day already in place.

Elaine and her parents pulled into the circular driveway and parked behind Al's 1957 black MG that a kind soul from the plant had made sure found its way home. Shocked, she first thought she had stepped back to reality from a surreal nightmare.

"Oh, my God." She started to cry and found she could not stop herself.

The driver's door opened and closed as her father exited the car wordlessly. She felt her mother's arms around her as Mrs. Hinds slid closer to her daughter in the back seat.

Words mixed with tears as Elaine lost the composure she fought so hard to maintain. "He'll never drive again, Mom. He loved that car. He always wanted to be a jet pilot. Did I ever tell you that?"

"Shhh. I know, I know." Mrs. Hinds held her daughter tightly. "He's alive. He's alive and he's a fighter. Always has been. You have a life with this man and that life is not over."

"How can I do this?" Elaine started to project on a dark future.

Mrs. Hinds replied, "Are you still married to the same man you met as a freshman in high school? You know him better than anyone. When has he made a compromise? When has he ever given up? He rolls with whatever is thrown at him and laughs. He finds a way to work with life and thrives on challenge. His favorite saying is, 'You either face life and find a way to enjoy yourself or lay down and die'. Now, from what I heard today, he is not going to die." Mrs. Hinds felt her own strength returning as she faced her young daughter.

"Mom, I'm scared." Elaine shook slightly.

"I know, but you will do whatever it takes. You always have. You are the reason Al chose to go to college instead of staying at his full, time construction job. Now as his wife you will fight through this together." Mrs. Hinds smiled weakly.

Unable to return the smile, Elaine stared blankly out the windshield of the station wagon, trying to make sense out of her mother's speech. "I guess I forgot the man I married. He is so helpless and in agony."

"Let him heal. Let him regain his strength." She knew she had gotten through to her daughter even if only in a small way. Elaine and Helen sat in the silence of the car's interior as nightfall gathered around them. Eventually, Elaine reached for the door handle, climbed out of the station wagon, passed the MG, and walked into the well-lit house.

Chapter IV: In the Sphere

*T*he first ten days of his hospital stay were lost to Al while he remained heavily medicated in the ICU. He was unaware of the emotional turmoil his family endured as each one struggled with the medical facts and logistics of his admittance to Overlook Hospital. Machines beeped, a steady stream of doctors, nurses and family came and went, but he was unaware of the activity. Intermittently conscious on the tenth day, Al realized, to his horror, that in addition to the agony he felt, he was also blind. Consumed with the pain and darkness that surrounded him, he did not immediately interact with anyone and instead carried on an internal monologue.

I can't do this, I can't do this. It's too much. What is that smell? It smells like burnt hamburger. My God, My God, I can't see.

The nurses brought the world back to him slowly. "Try to relax, Mr. Plevier. You need to work within the pain medication we administer." The nurse placed a needle in Al's arm, injecting him with encroaching oblivion.

The pain relented into numbness as his mind began to drift.

"I unt ooo eee. Laine?" Absent of lips, his words sounded senseless.

Al fell into dreamless oblivion and was rudely brought back to reality. The pain in his head and burning of his skin made him cry out in protest.

"Oooo."

"Mr. Plevier? You need to wake up. It's time to clean your mouth. Mr. Plevier? You've been out for several hours." The nurse would not give up until Al fought through the haze of painkillers that were his refuge. He groaned and tried to turn his head. "I understand, but you're never going to get out of here unless we work together. You have a long way to go, but you can do it." Al turned his head to the nurse and she gently went about the business of rinsing his brutalized mouth. "You're doing great. Today is October 11, around six o'clock in the morning."

The smell of burnt meat had been assaulting Al's senses since awakening. "Wat da sell?" Al hoped the nurse could understand his meaning through his disintegrated lips and tortured internal mouth.

The nurse raised her eyebrows with surprise. "I'm not sure what you smell, but with the extent of your injuries, it's great to know that you can smell."

Al formed his own conclusion. "Is it EE?"

The nurse looked at the man turning his head toward her. "You experienced burns to all layers of the skin in the areas that had contact with the sodium hydroxide. The damage was 60 percent of your body and the odor from the burned tissue and flesh might linger."

I'll never eat a hamburger again. Someone should stick a fork in me and consider me done. Al tried to find a waft of air somewhere inside the room that would relieve him from the torturous smell.

The nurse applied medication to the remnants of the lips Elaine had thought no longer existed. After she finished, the stale taste of collateral damage returned to him.

"Time for breakfast." The nurse tried to change the subject

as she checked his feeding tube and replaced an empty bag with another containing more life sustaining nourishment.

What is in my mouth? She must have left something in there. My tongue feels like leather. Not even the rinse helped.

Al ran his tongue over the roof of his mouth. Something dislodged and promptly spit it out onto his chin.

The nurse looked up from the tray she now worked over. "Did I leave something behind, dear? Let me see." She bent closer and looked over the object resting on his chin. "I need to look into your mouth. You spit out a piece of your palate." She wiped the flesh from his chin and reached for a small flashlight.

This is gross. That chemical's not done with me yet. It's gonna keep going until it dissolves me and goes right through the net I'm lying on. At least it feels like a net. Maybe a hammock.

"Mr. Plevier, are you ready for your codeine?"

Is she kidding me? I can't see. I can only feel pain.

A few seconds later the drug took effect. He awakened the second time that day it was to Elaine's voice he heard. "I'm here, Al."

"Ane?"

"Yes, it's me." She leaned toward him. "I love you." Elaine could not hold her husband's hand and still had to be dressed in the protective visitor's clothing. Behind the plastic tent that hung over him, she could see the face of the man she loved trying to reshape itself as the swelling slowly receded. "Everyone at home is fine so don't worry about us. Just get well. We want you home." Feeling the weight of the baby growing inside her, Elaine sat down next to Al's bed in the chair the nurse had brought for her. She kept the one-sided conversation going with topics that gave her weary spirits a lift. "I had a doctor's appointment for a regular checkup and heard the baby's heartbeat."

The baby, Little Albert, Elaine. I have to get out of here.

Elaine didn't know if Al believed her measures of his healing progress on her visits, but she didn't see the harm in continuing. "Some of the swelling in your face has decreased."

What does that matter to me? I can't see.

(42)

"Albert picked up that baseball you got him, tossed it and said, Daddy." Elaine heard Al make a small sound. "He really did. I told him you would be home soon"

A dialogue of self, pity started inside his head. *To do what? I can't throw a ball to my kid anymore. What kind of a father will I be?*

"I'll let you know if I leave the room. I'll be taking a walk while the nurse works on you." Elaine reached into her pocket for something the doctor said was permitted to bring into the ICU. "Aunt Catherine sent this scapular the night of the accident. I wasn't allowed to bring it in until now." Elaine stared at the two small plastic slips that held pictures of the Sacred Heart and the Blessed Mother. She draped the piece of twelve- inch yarn that was strung between them over the knob on the wall intercom. "I hung the scapular behind your head."

" 'aine."

"Yes. I'm still here. You rest. I should still be here the next time you wake up."

Al began to relax into his pain, knowing Elaine was nearby. *Thank you, God, for letting me live. Our Father...*

Al fell back into drug assisted oblivion before he finished praying. The next thing he knew he was abruptly awakened to an almost full mental state of alertness. The burns on the right side of his chest seared through him as hands moved over his body. Someone was cleaning and tearing off the burned, dead skin.

"Mr. Plevier, are you with us? Try to relax as we clean your wounds. This is the debridement procedure that you have usually been sedated during. I know it's painful. We have to remove the dead skin or you run the risk of an infection."

Two nurses worked on Al. He was rolled first to his left and then to his right as he lay on the mesh netting. With the plastic covering and blanket that usually laid over his body pulled back, he felt cold.

He cried out, unashamed and unembarrassed. "Ou! Sto!"

The debridement procedure normally lasted for about thirty minutes. The skin removed was dead, but the nerves were not. It left him physically and mentally exhausted.

The doctors have my body and God has my soul. This is a nightmare. I need drugs for this. I'm gonna die while I'm peeled.

The procedure ended as unceremoniously as it started. "We're finished, Mr. Plevier. We've given you something that will help you rest. You'll be ready for the upgrade to Isolation soon."

While in ICU Al had no concept of night or day. For an upgrade to Isolation, he would begin to be weaned on the dosage of the pain medication protocol and placed into a regular sleeping schedule to begin his discernment of the passage time as a blind individual. A patient in Isolation must be kept from other patients to prevent the chance of infection but requires less monitoring and attention than a patient in ICU.

Toward the end of his stay in ICU, the reduction in Al's pain medications allowed for longer periods of lucidity and clarity. These periods of time were accompanied by the intense pain of his healing burns that he had to learn to manage and work within. On day seventeen, he was prepped for the move to Isolation. Fear gripped Al as the unknown loomed in front of him.

I don't even know what time of the day it is. I can't see. I need someone with me all the time. How can I function outside the walls of this room? What do I look like? I'm still in constant pain. I need my medication.

Al heard someone approach his bedside. "You must be happy to be one step closer to home." The nurse tried to sound cheerful.

I'll be one more kid for Elaine to take care of. How will I ever make it out there?

"I'll give you something to help you sleep when we get to your new room. I know you are in discomfort, but we want you alert for the move."

Dr. Westmont entered the room unannounced. "Good morning, Albert. How are you today?"

Is he serious? "Ine."

"Today is a big deal. Your progress is steady. We want to get you back on your feet. If this had happened to anyone else, I'd

(44)

keep them here longer. You've had your age and health on your side to help you fight. You have a lot to be thankful for." Dr. Westmont looked over the chart in his hand and wrote comments as he spoke.

This guy is *serious.* "Ow uch longer?"

"A couple of minutes. Your speech is improving. I know it must be uncomfortable."

"hanks."

As Dr. Westmont spoke, Al could hear papers rustling. "I need to prepare you for a few things."

Prepare me for what? Are you going cut out my liver while I'm conscious? What is left for you to torture me with? "Wha nes?"

A male nurse spoke to Dr. Westmont from the doorway. "Are you ready Doctor?"

"Yes, I think so. I was about to brief Albert." Dr. Westmont waited for the two nurses to leave the room. "Al this will be your first impression of the outside world after the relative security of these four walls. You will have a lot of input to your other senses. Do you have any questions?" The doctor continued. "One blessing in your accident is that none of the chemicals seeped into your ear canals. That would have meant a permanent hearing loss, brain damage or death. Your hearing will actually be heightened."

Great. Al lay on his mesh netting, wondering how he could ask questions not knowing what to expect next. "I'm ood."

I want to stay here a little longer. Please don't move me yet. I'm not ready.

"The nurses will wheel you to your room and I'll meet you there." Dr. Westmont left without any further conversation.

Al heard footsteps around his bed. "We're ready Sir."

The move out of the room that had become both a prison and a sanctuary to Al started slowly as he felt his body being lifted off the mesh netting and transferred to a movable bed. The feel of the solid mattress under him was both shocking and painful. No longer under a tent sheet, he felt a light material being draped over his body. The plastic cover that had been tented over the bed for

(45)

protection was now removed permanently.

People worked around him and then he felt the bed move. The forward motion caught him by surprise, and he found himself gripping both sides of the bed for fear of rolling out. He was unable to know that the orderlies and nurse were still wearing protective clothing and gloves. Isolation would still be for his protection.

What do I look like to everyone else? I hope someone had the brains to cover me with a dark colored blanket. I don't want anyone looking at me. At least the doctors and the nurses understand someone that is banged up like me. I want to have some dignity. This doctor thinks he is moving me to isolation, but I'm already living in isolation.

The bed was turned all the way to the right to make the sharp turn out the doorway. As the bed moved forward, it gathered pace.

He was sure it was moving too fast. "o own. Sooo own!"

"Try to stay calm. You're safe. This is a new sensation for you." The nurses slowed the bed slightly but needed to move forward and not have Al in the corridors for too long.

He could hear footsteps moving past the bed in the corridor. *Life really does go on without you.* Desperately Al tried to go inside his own head and pretend he was somewhere else. *I hope no one is staring. Someone should have pulled the sheet over my head for the trip. Why is there so much noise? How many phones does a hospital have? And what is that smell? I can feel breezes as people walk by. I wonder if the world knows how fast their lives are moving? Everyone is racing back and forth. How can people not bump into each other?* Listening to the clips of conversation and fast-moving feet, Al suddenly wished he were among 'the others'.

"Mr. Plevier, in a minute we will be entering the elevator. First, we will make a left at the end of the hall." The soft, melodic, practiced tone of the details, conveyed an experience she possessed in her field that betrayed her age. "The new room will be quieter." I bet you'll be glad to be in a different environment."

(46)

Unless I'm home, it's all the same to me, Lady.

"Sow own. Eez. Too fas. Too fas." Panic gripped Al as the bed turned left.

"We're sorry, Mr. Plevier. We'll try to go as slow as we can." The male nurse apologized, but didn't know how to explain to the blind man on his gurney that the bed was almost creeping along the corridor.

The more experienced nurse chimed in to calm Al's fears. "It's all the sensory input you are receiving. You've been in your bed in ICU for two weeks without movement. Without sight, your hearing and your equilibrium are overloaded leaving you feeling like a visitor in the middle of an alien city."

I'm the alien. I don't belong here. Everyone is probably looking at the poor bastard being wheeled down the hall. I must look like road kill. I don't want to be here.

The first trip outside the sheltered environment of ICU left him unprepared for his new interpretation of life. The consolation was that the excursion drew his attention away from the constant pain and discomfort.

"We're at the elevator." The nurse looked at her patient with a worried look that she hoped was not conveyed in her voice. "How are you doing?"

"Ine." Al commented quickly.

If I don't throw up in this thing it will be a miracle. I want to go back to my old room. Maybe I should never leave. There's no way I can cope in the outside world.

The doors to the elevator opened, and before Al could protest the bed rolled over the doorway grooves. He was inside and the doors were closing. The elevator dipped slightly and then began its ascent. Al rolled his head to one side trying to stabilize his mind.

Whoa. I need to throw up. "I'm onna ee ick." He continued to hold the bedrails in a deathgrip.

The nurses were patient and held a small receptacle next to the bed. "If you feel you are going to throw up we'll roll you to the side."

(47)

Multiple external stimuli assaulted his senses beginning with a ringing phone immediately to his left. The blips of conversations blended into one continuous dialogue of nonsense. "How did you... move the man over... hurry to ICU...not today...lunch was a struggle with my new diet...I can't find...Mr. Plevier how are you doing...never again...Dr. Caroly... to emergency...the baby was four pounds..."

The continuous soft rolling of the wheels underneath the bed was a comfort amidst what Al considered to be the pandemonium around him. Thoughts ran quickly through his mind.

If I could relax maybe the sound of the wheels would put me to sleep. What is that constant humming? It's not one of my machines. It sounds like it's over my head. It never leaves no matter where I travel. Those intercoms should be turned down. There's just too much noise. I wish Elaine were here. I need her to be my eyes and tell me what is going on. I don't think these guys are being careful enough. If the bed bumps into something, I could fall right off.

Al felt the bed make a right turn and then come to a crawl as the attendants turned the stretcher wide. Without any grandeur, the journey ended.

"Mr. Plevier we're in your new room. Let's get you settled and then we'll give you something to let you sleep for a few hours." The nurses moved the bed around in the room until it was positioned exactly as it needed to be. Al could feel the nurse checking the IV line he was transported with and the catheter. "Your lines are good. You should have the catheter out soon. I have an oral sedative in liquid form to relax you."

"Anks." Al was very still as he desperately tried to hide and calm the fear paralyzing his confidence.

The nurse raised his bed and he sipped the liquid through a straw. Now on a new floor in a new room at the far end of the corridor away from the nurses' station. No one would be passing by on their way to check on another patient. Without TV or radio to ease the prolonged hours of uninterrupted silence that enveloped him isolation was truly isolating. He tried to empty his mind and allow the medication to take effect. He could not stop thinking about his family.

He began to reorient his thoughts toward the positive.

Elaine and I will get through this. I know it in my heart. I have faith in both of us. Our marriage is solid. Albert is happy and healthy. I'm alive. I don't care who is in front of me or who is in back of me, as long as I'm still in the human race. I just need to regain my strength. I have to find a reference point. I won't quit on my family.

Al's mind began to spin as he thought about his inability to work.

I've been working since I was eight, delivering papers for the twelve- year old on the block, who took a cut. I can do this. Starting over is a chance to do it better. We still have our real estate money to fall back on. We can do this.

The last visual image Al had in his mind's eye was of Elaine holding Albert. He then entered into the narcotic-induced oblivion without dreams.

Chapter V: Improvisation

*C*oping with recovery and the loneliness of Isolation allowed for the removal of the protective plastic tent and, to his surprise, the catheter. He was given a urine receptacle, but told to call a nurse for assistance. The first two days Al was visited by a nurse only for the disbursement of medication, assistance elimination needs, or to have his wounds cleaned during the debridement procedure. His room at the end of the hall offered little opportunity for a nurse to observe him while on her way to the room of another patient. Elaine brought a small radio for Al that he kept on all day and night with the volume very low. She felt that the location of the room was not a suitable arrangement for a man with injuries as extensive as Al had sustained even though he still needed contact protection. She asked the doctor and nurses every day for a room change. Additionally, he was no longer on the regulated sleeping schedule established during his ICU stay. Day and night interchanged.

Between the doses of pain medication, he began to absorb the parameters of his new life. The darkness was not a monster, or even a fearful reality, it was a new way to learn to live. In a moment of clarity, it became obvious to him that living without sight was going to be a pain-in-the-ass.

On the twentieth day of his hospitalization at eleven in the morning, Al reached to his left, felt along the bed rail where the call button would be clipped and rang for a nurse. After what seemed like an eternity, he pushed the button. Two more attempts and he knew he was alone.

Anxiety grew with each attempt. He wondered where the nurse on duty was.

What is going on? I need someone. Are the nurses all on a coffee break? Why wasn't the catheter left in if they aren't going to help with the receptacle?

Panic grew and Al yelled out in frustration. "Hey!" He felt the reverberation in his lungs and throat. As he waited one thought was prominent in his mind.

This is no good.

Al's heart began to race as he became more frustrated and frightened.

I can't help myself. This is no good. I'm alone down here.

He tried to attract the attention of a nurse for another ten minutes, yelling as loud as he could. "Eez! Where are you? I nee hel own ere. Hey!" Finally, he gave up.

He decided to devise a new strategy that felt more like a plan for survival than calling the nurse's station. Using his left arm, he began to reach where he knew the movable table on wheels was located. On top of the table were various items used during the day to take care of Al. He grabbed the edge of the table and with what strength he had, lifted its edge and shoved as hard as he could. It landed with a bang and clatter as the metals pans scattered and rolled onto the linoleum square tiles that made up the hospital room floor.

Instantly, Al heard the ding of patient buzzers going off down the corridor and he smirked derisively as he thought about his success. *At least I got someone's attention.* It was then that he realized he never heard any sound coming from his own call button.

The fast padding of nurse's shoes approached his door. "Mr. Plevier, what is going on in here?" The nurse looked at the overturned table. "How did you manage that?"

(51)

Al tried to control his anger, knowing how badly he needed the nurse, and how it still hurt to speak through his healing lips. "I ave een ringing and ringing or u. Ere er you?"

The nurse bent down to begin cleaning the mess. "You have not been ringing your bell. Someone would have come immediately." She righted the table and stood next to his bed. "You do not have to be so nasty. We're here to help you."

Al used all his self-restraint not to scream. "I'm telling you. I ave een trying to cawl you."

The nurse bent over to pick up some of the items, placed them back on the table and then looked down at Al. "Your buzzer is next to your left hand, still clipped to the bed rail. No more tantrums. At least save them for the next shift. Now, what is it that you need?"

Al felt like a helpless child. "I need to ee."

The impatient nurse responded quickly. "Fine. Let's take care of you and then try to relax." She moved around the room tending to Al's needs and turned with one last instruction. "Remember, no tantrums."

Al heard her shoes retreating down the hallway. He began to devise a plan. *Fine. I can't lie here waiting for the next problem and no one to help me. I'll deal with this myself.*

First Al tried to ring the buzzer and did not hear the ding he had heard from other patients' rooms. He held the buzzer in his right hand, traced it with his left, found the place where the cord clipped to the bed, unclipped it and yanked. Not to his surprise, the cord flew into his lap.

Either this thing requires no effort at all to pull out of the wall or it was never plugged in. Maybe the cleaning people knocked it out. Whatever. It doesn't matter. I'm fixing this myself. Enough.

In severe pain, Al lowered the side of his bed with his left hand. It required him to lift up and push the rail forward and down. He paused after this effort to catch his breath and rest from the pain. The bed was raised only two feet off the ground, allowing him to ease his body onto his left side, slip off the mattress, and let

(52)

his feet touch the floor. This was the first time since the accident that his legs held him and they both shook responsively. His weight had dropped to 130 pounds from a pre-accident of 164 and consequently, he felt each precarious movement he made. Squatting beside the bed, holding on to the edge to steady himself, he briefly thought he should reconsider what the hell he was doing before continuing.

Screw it. I have to take care of myself.

He crouched next to his bed and felt around on the floor breathing heavily through the pain in both his body and behind his eyes. Moving forward a few inches he ran his left hand over the wall behind the headboard until he found the electrical socket about a foot off the floor. Stopping for a few seconds to think through what to do next, he found himself gripping the cord more tightly than necessary creating intense pain in his severely damaged right hand.

At least I can feel.

Still crouching and grasping the cord in his right hand while he leaned his body against the bed, he found the end of the call button line. He bent down, with his burned skin tearing with each movement he made and plugged the cord into the wall. Squeezing the button, he felt the muscles in his hand react more painfully as the accompanying ding of his own buzzer reached his ears.

I win.

The dinging of the button brought a smile to Al's face as the padded shoes he heard before were now accompanied by a gasp. "Oh, my God! What do you think you're doing?" The horrified nurse rushed to Al, crouching naked next to his bed. Unable to touch the right side of his body that he exposed to her, she bent over him and reached around to his left shoulder and gently tried to coax him toward the bed behind him. "Give me that buzzer!" With her left hand, she took the object of contempt from Al's still clutching right hand. "You're going to be lucky if you haven't done more damage to yourself."

Slowly, Al and the nurse managed to get him back to bed

with his knees bent and right arm cradled. The nurse raised the side of the bed, clicking the railing into place. "If you ever pull a stunt like that again, I swear I will tie you to this bed. I'm telling the doctor to order a psych exam on you. Time will tell if you've set yourself back in your recovery time." The nurse clipped the buzzer to the rail and placed the button in Al's left hand. "What possessed you to do that and how the hell did you ever get out of bed and lower the side rail?"

Al couldn't believe what he heard. *Is she kidding me?* "Are you kidding ee? The uzzer lug was oudda the wall. You didn eleive ee. Whadda sect ee to do, lie here and die?"

The nurse instantly felt bad. "You're set now. Maybe I should also ask the doctor to lower your painkillers. That should keep you from pulling any more stunts like this. And by the way, your speech is getting better every day. I know it hurts to talk." The nurse turned to leave the room. "I'll be back shortly to make sure you're behaving."

"I'll ee waiting…" Al heard her retreating shoes. After he was sure she moved down the corridor, he laughed out loud for the first time in three weeks.

I'm going to be all right.

Chapter VI: Polarities

Al slept soundly for the rest of the morning with the radio lulling him into restful oblivion. He awakened when Elaine arrived at three.

"Hi, Al. How are you?" She made herself as comfortable in the protective gown and gloves she was still required to wear.

"laine, I ha an interesting orning." Al smiled, which considering the condition of his healing lips, looked mostly like a grimace.

"Let's have it." Elaine sat down heavily in the chair trying to relax the tension the pregnancy was adding to her lower back.

Just as Al was about to speak, the same nurse who earlier found him crouched next to his bed walked into the room. "Did he tell you what he did today?"

Elaine turned her attention to the nurse. "No. He was about to."

"Apparently, we had trouble with the call button and your husband decided to climb out of bed and fix it himself." The nurse crossed her arms for effect.

"You had trouble with the call button? Did you try to fix it before him?" The tension in Elaine's body returned.

"We didn't realize there was a problem." The nurse stuttered slightly when she saw Elaine's face harden.

"Until what? He fixed it himself? Are you kidding me? How long did it take for you to realize what he was doing?" She let the anger rise and release some of the tension in her back.

The nurse paused with a red face before responding. "I found him on the floor next to the bed."

"What!" Elaine got up out of the chair to face the nurse.

While he listened to the two women, Al lay quiet and satisfied in his bed. If he could have smirked, he would.

"First of all, you have a critically injured man at the end of the hall, which in and of itself is ridiculous. Second, he had enough time alone to get out of his bed and fix a buzzer. He could have laid here for hours if he needed you. I want him moved closer to the nurses' desk now. Not tomorrow, not in several hours, now!"

The nurse, somewhat shocked by the bold side to Elaine's personality, turned and left the room.

"If she isn't back here in twenty minutes with two orderlies, I'll take care of this myself." Elaine moved about the room gathering up Al's few possessions and then dropped into the chair next to his bed, staring at the clock over his door.

Al wanted to reach out and wrap his arms around his wife. "Aane, tha was grea."

"We'll get you out of here." She felt the tension of the last three weeks flowing out of her. "Please, don't do anything that stupid again."

The original nurse, still red faced, and two orderlies entered the room. "Mr. Plevier, you're going to be moved to a room across from the nursing station."

Elaine called Workmen's Compensation Insurance to discuss what had happened and was informed that Al was entitled to a private duty nurse twenty-four-hours a day due to the extent of his injuries. The next day Al was introduced to Mary for the day shift and Jack for the night shift. Jack was an angel of mercy, but Mary was a constant source of antagonism whom Al referred to privately as the bitch from hell.

The first night of Jack's duty, itching from the healing skin of the burned tissue combined with the pain became unbearable. Jack was the first person who brought Al relief from a source other than drugs.

"Mr. Plevier, I brought my spoons with me tonight." Jack wasted no time opening the black bag he brought with him.

The tinkling sound of silverware resounded in Al's ears. "Huh?" Al couldn't imagine what the nurse was talking about.

Jack began to instruct his patient. "Roll onto your left side as much as you can." Jack lifted the gown Al wore.

Before Al knew what was happening, he felt the cool relief of smooth metal running over his back. "Ahhh. Thanks. Ahhh." The relief he felt made the urgency for the pain relief medication drift away. "Can we do this every night?"

Jack looked compassionately at Al. "Yes. That's my job." He watched as Al deeply relaxed into the procedure. "We can couple this with your saline baths. I'll have to speak to the day shift to see if we can switch your bath schedule over to my night shift. If not, I'll sneak you in."

Al gave a low laugh directed toward Jack. "Good luck wid dat. It's like being in the army here."

On the third night of Jack's duty, in the middle of his spooning session, he stopped abruptly and awakened Al, who had drifted to sleep from the soothing procedure combined with light medication. "Al, wake up, I pulled some strings to get you a night bath. You'll have privacy."

Al became fully awake. "Do I get my bath tonight?"

Jack worked to finish the spoon procedure as he spoke to Al. "Yes. You can enjoy your saline bath alone tonight instead of wondering who else is in the room. I have to finish the chores Mary left for me and get you ready to be moved." Jack rolled Al gently onto his back and pulled the blanket over him.

He listened and followed every movement Jack made. *He's moving aside all the dirty linens Mary left behind. He's collecting the garbage she left. He's checking my wounds. It must have been thirty minutes already. I don't know how this miracle was allowed but, I wish we would get going before someone changes their mind.*

After what seemed like an eternity to Al, Jack spoke. "Let's move you downstairs." He waited for a response from Al. "Am I losing you to sleep before I get you downstairs?"

"Are you nus? I thought you never finish. You took forever picking up the laundry and garbage Mary left for you."

Jack stopped in his tracks before speaking. "You knew I picked up the laundry? That's great. You're paying more attention to the world. That's a natural transition and a good thing since you're going to be living in it sooner than you think."

Jack lifted Al into the wheelchair that he was now permitted to use. The chair was uncomfortable, but he preferred it the hospital bed. Sitting upright gave him the proper perspective on the environment and allowed him to interact with his immediate world. Jack wheeled him steadily down the empty corridor.

He shifted a tiny bit in the chair. "I can't wait to get down there. I don't even mind the elevator anymore."

Jack gave a broad, friendly smile, and hoped his voice conveyed that to Al. "I know. The chair is a nice graduation from the bed." The elevator dinged and he gently turned the chair around and pulled Al through the doors. "I hooked you up with the same therapist you had for your baths during the day. He's a nice kid and understands where you are in your healing process. Pain and itching at the same time can make a person ask for more drugs instead of learning how to work through the pain."

Al turned his head gratefully toward Jack. "Thanks, Jack." He shifted in the chair as the burns and his normal nervous tick reacted together.

During the bath, the therapist would immerse Al's battered body into water that was slightly warmer than body temperature. He would first be placed on a firm mesh and then lifted into the tub by a set of pulleys and ropes. During the day, other people were in the room and Al was never sure who was watching his naked body being eased into the baths. Tonight, it was just Al, Jack and a physical therapist.

Soon the short elevator ride was over. Al felt the familiar, lift-drop before the doors opened. The change in the air confirmed for him that he was near the physical therapy area.

Danny, the therapist, yelled a greeting to him. "Hi, Mr. Plevier. It's Danny from the afternoon shift."

Al smiled as he recalled internally who was speaking to him. *Nice kid. At least tonight I don't have to wonder who else is watching my naked ass.* Al shook his head and laugh out loud as the therapist and nurse exchanged puzzled looks.

Jack lifted Al into the net and Danny worked the pullies to ease his body into the warm water. "Ahhh... Can I do this every night?" Al had high hopes that this would put him on a schedule of sleeping during Mary's shift.

Jack stepped back to let Danny do his job. "I'm working on it."

The protective, supportive mesh net he laid on offered the security a person without sight relied on. Each ripple of water reverberated over his skin and was felt by the remaining, raw, damaged nerve endings. Exhaustion and anger began to rise inside his head as the water worked for and a little against him.

Isn't it bad enough I'm blind? I can live with that, somehow. I don't know if I can live with the dark and pain. I just want to sleep it off. I just want to sleep forever.

Jack watched Al closely and saw his body relax. He appeared to be asleep. "Al, come on. Stay with us." Jack watched and felt Al staying inside his own head longer than usual.

Al shook himself fully awake and then let Jack know he was alert. "All I ant to do is slee as I lie in this ater. The relief is onderful."

"Come on, Al. Just a few more minutes in the saline so we can have a complete session. Your wife tells me your speech is improving. I know it stills hurts your lips, but you're healing perfectly." Al didn't respond and Jack knew he had timed the bath perfectly and that Al would now sleep through the night possibly without the aid of narcotics.

After the bath, he was already asleep for the return trip and did not awaken as Jack lifted him into the hospital bed. Al slept so soundly that he never heard Jack leave. The next morning around eight he heard the voices of a young nurse and Mary the day shift nurse from Workmen's Compensation who had never dressed in the required protective clothing for Isolation.

Mary saw Al begin to stir. "Good morning Mr. Plevier. We have a nice long morning ahead of us until your wife gets here." Mary smiled at the bandaged eyes in front of her.

Al felt a sense of dread spread over him. "Hello ary. You're early. Husband throw you out?" He had survived four day shifts under Mary's care and hoped biting comments would make her want to quit.

Mary moved about the small room doing little to care for Al. She moved to the far windowless wall to look over the cards from the friends and family. After reading through them, she dropped into her chair and watched the clock as it moved closer to noon and Elaine's arrival.

"Mr. Plevier, wake up." Al had tried in vain to pretend to drift back to sleep. "You know you're not supposed to sleep during the day." She stood and walked over to the bedside, leaning over Al's face, her large breasts squishing against the bed rail. "Come on, you have new cards for us to look at together. I can read them to you." Satisfied that he was fully awake, Mary plopped back down into the chair. "I don't know who this person Sam is, but he only spent twenty-five cents on your card." She dropped the first on the table and held the second. "This person spent fifty cents. I guess you rank a little higher in his social ladder."

A doctor entered the room as Mary held the third card. "Hello, Albert."

Al baited Mary while the doctor was present. "Aren't you going to keep reading my cards to me?"

The middle-aged doctor looked Mary up and down. "Where are your gown and gloves?" Mary ignored the doctor and walked out of the room leaving him to shake his head in disgust.

"Good morning Albert, it's Dr. Euclid. How are you today?" The doctor picked up Al's medical chart.

"I know who you are. You don't have to keep telling me."

Al relaxed a little with Mary's absence. "When can I eave?"

Dr. Euclid laughed as he continued looking over the chart. "You'll be out of here sooner than you think. I bet you'll even miss us."

"Doc, I won't iss ary. You have got to get me a new nurse. She's crazy. I can't take one ore day with her." Al knew he sounded desperate, but what he didn't realize was that Mary had walked back into the room.

Dr. Euclid caught her look of fury as she grabbed the bag she had forgotten and walked back out. "Albert, she was just here. I'm afraid you've made a bad enemy out of the wicked witch of the west."

Al groaned. "She can't ee any orse than she already is."

Dr. Euclid sat with Al for fifteen minutes longer than usual discussing where he felt Al was in his recovery. He had been in the hospital for twenty-four days and both men were ready to gamble on the possibility of a release date if his progress continued as well as it had been. Al hoped in his heart that he would be home with his family for Thanksgiving.

It wasn't long after the doctor left that Al heard Mary's heavy padding as she entered his hospital room. His hands began to shake. *Damn.*

She walked over to Al's bed and leaned down next to his ear, her warm breath saturated with coffee and cigarettes. "You think you need a new nurse?" Mary, still not dressed in protective clothing, stood straight and reached to her left to arrange the instruments she had carried in.

Al breathed in and tried to steady his nerves. *Kill me now God.* He could hear Mary preparing her medical instruments. "Are you getting ready for my debridement, ary? What a'out the drugs?"

Mary continued with her work, acting as if she never heard Al. "Yes, it's time for your debridement. Are you ready, dear?" She turned on the portable radio Al kept next to the bed and raised the volume.

Al tried not to stutter as he reminded Mary about the drugs

(61)

usually given to him during the debridement procedure. "Mary, where are the drugs to knock ee out?" Al felt the light blanket and sheet pulled away from his body. Out of habit he slowly rolled to his left side.

The debridement procedure for Al was a dreaded experience, but today he was terrified. The pain that occurs as the dead tissue is peeled away from the healing tissue underneath and then cleansed is unavoidable.

Mary lowered the side of the bed. "You're strong enough now to stand up as I move through the debridement." She left Al to climb out of the bed on his own. "If you climbed out of bed to fix your buzzer four days ago, you can handle this. Be quick about it. I have a tight schedule."

Al climbed carefully out of bed and stood upright and slightly bent over, not knowing what to do next.

Seeing his hesitation, Mary barked orders at him. "Stand facing the wall to your left. I moved the table and your wife's chair already." Mary had rolled the table to where she could easily reach her instruments.

Al began to shake and was worried that his legs would not hold him. *This woman is out of her mind. If I live through this she has to go.* He lifted his left arm, felt the wall and leaned into it. Without any warning, Mary opened the back of his gown completely and began to peel the skin.

Instantly, the pain seared through Al. "Owwwww!"

Mary smiled. "Let me do my job. The quicker I work the sooner this will be over." Ironically, the faster Mary worked the longer it took.

Five minutes into the treatment, Al lost control. "You're a crazy bitch!"

Mary laughed out loud. "That came out nice and clear didn't it? We have a lot more skin to peel. Try to relax." Her face became animated as she became focused on torturing Al. "If you want to leave this place and be as healthy as can be expected under the circumstances, you need to get rid of that dead, rotting skin. It

(62)

does start to smell. I mean, really, do you think the dead, burnt, useless, smelly skin is going to flake off by itself? You are not normal anymore." Mary smiled broadly and never noticed the floor nurse standing silently behind her in the doorway.

The floor nurse, summoned by the loud radio, could not believe what she was seeing. "What is going on in here?" The head floor nurse looked with horror at the smile on Mary's face, Al standing against the wall for a procedure usually done lying down, and Mary not wearing surgical scrubs or gloves. "I'll finish Mr. Plevier's procedure. Go take a walk, Mary."

"No, I don't think so. I'm the private duty nurse and I'm in charge of this patient." Mary's smile broadened.

The two women squared off as Al leaned heavily against the wall. The face of the head floor nurse's demeanor turned to granite. "I'm sure with one call to Mrs. Plevier, you'll be relieved. Go find something to do while I finish this patient's debridement." The head nurse brushed past Mary and continued gently with Al. "Mr. Plevier. Let's get this over with and get you back to bed." Mary walked out, staring over her shoulder with disdain and fury as the floor nurse kept eye contact with her until Mary walked through the open door. "She won't be back, Mr. Plevier. I'll call Dr. Euclid, your wife, and the board to complain. I knew there was something else wrong with her beyond her miserable disposition. She's dangerous."

Al felt his body begin to relax. "Thanks." He didn't make another sound during the rest of the gentler, but still painful procedure.

Weakened by the ordeal, the nurse helped Al back into bed and gave him a narcotic that allowed him to fall immediately into a fitful sleep. He awoke the familiar smell of the perfume Elaine always wore was in the room. "Elaine?"

"I'm here Al. How are you?" Elaine reached over to touch her husband's left hand and felt the clamminess in his palm.

"Not good. You have to get rid of ary. She's not just a bitch, she's crazy. She tried to kill me this morning." Al began to roll onto his back from the stationary position he maintained on his

(63)

left side.

"The head nurse caught me on the way in here and told me what happened. I'll call Worker's Compensation while I'm here and arrange for a new nurse. If this is not possible for the day shift tomorrow, you may be without a private duty day nurse for that one shift. I can't believe you had to endure her on top of everything else." Elaine angrily tossed the magazine she read while Al had been sleeping.

"I just glad she'll ee gone. I can live with that." He breathed deeply. "Thank God for Jack. I feel normal with him."

Elaine watched Al's scarred face relaxing. "I spoke to Dr. Euclid on the phone after you talked to him this morning. According to him and Dr. Westmont, you've now been upgraded to Intermediate care. You'll stay in the same room. How is that for normal?" Elaine rubbed her stomach as she adjusted herself in the chair. "I hope those two are right and that you really will be home by Thanksgiving."

"I'm counting on it." Al heard his stomach rumble. "Did you bring me a milkshake today?" Al reached for the button to adjust his bed.

"I have it right here." Elaine opened the bag she had with her and pulled out the liquid McDonald's vanilla milkshake. "Sorry, it liquified. I've been here a while." She pressed it into his left hand. "Keep eating these and you'll be back to 164 pounds before you know it."

He carefully put the straw in his mouth in the most comfortable position and took a long sip. "Jack said I'm 130 last night. I never thought I would ee this skinny. It's scary." The smell of pizza wafted into the room as Al finished his second drag of milkshake. "God, that sells great. I'd love a iece."

"I'll see if the nurses can spare a slice." Elaine came back carrying a slice of pizza cut into four sections. "Let's see how you do with this. Be careful with your lips." She lifted Al's left hand and placed one of the small pieces into it. Carefully he placed the piece past his lips and before chewing, sucked gently on the dough, enjoying the flavor for the first time since before the accident. He ate all four sections and felt full with satisfaction.

"Thanks, sweetheart." Al sat quietly with Elaine listening to the radio and toward the end of the afternoon fell asleep.

Elaine had left and Jack was on duty. "Mr. Plevier. I thought we agreed that you were not to sleep too during the day."

Al yawned satisfactorily and felt a tearing along his lips. "Sorry, Jack." Jack was ready immediately with a cloth.

"Be careful. You're feeling much better now and it's easy to forget that you still have to work within the boundaries of your healing skin." Jack finished patting the spots of blood off Al's new lips. "Speaking of boundaries, I heard that you had pizza this afternoon. You have to remember that you need to introduce foods slowly into your diet. I understand how good that must have tasted, but you should be eating the bland hospital food your doctor recommends. Don't go crazy in the beginning or it will not work out well for you." Jack laughed a little at the end of his lecture.

Al turned his head toward the nurse. "Jack, for you that was an evil laugh. What do you mean?"

"You'll throw up. You've been through a major trauma. Allow your body some adjustment time. You're doing great, but you are in your third week of recovery." Jack paused for effect. "Three weeks after a life-threatening accident is not very long. Surviving alone was a miracle." Jack sat and opened a book to begin reading to Al.

Al held up his left arm. "Jack, I'm too skinny. I can feel it. I must look like a skeleton."

Jack looked compassionately at his patient and then smirked. "From what your wife tells me, you were never much to look at before the weight loss buddy, so let's work through this."

Al snorted in agreement. "You're a funny man, Jack. Real funny."

"I brought a book about great sports legends to read to you." Jack pulled the book out of his bag.

"That's great. A book that finally holds my interest." Al stayed awake most of the night, unable to independently return to a normal sleeping pattern. When Mary's replacement arrived, she

(65)

was told by Jack, to keep Al awake.

"He needs to get into a normal sleeping pattern. Have them take him down for his saline bath in the afternoon. That should knock him out for the night." Jack looked at his patient.

Al jumped into the conversation between Jack and the new day nurse. "I'm blind, not deaf. Do I get a say in this?"

The two nurses answered him in unison. "No."

Al fought all morning to stay awake and managed to eat all the hospital food offered to him for breakfast. At eleven o'clock visiting hours started, and he began to feel nauseous.

The day nurse left the room to get supplies and an old High School friend of both Al and Elaine's came by for a visit. "Al, its Bob Kay."

"Hi, Bob." Al promptly threw up.

"Whoah!" Bob dropped the bag of food he had brought for Al on the table. "I'll get a nurse." Bob grabbed a small plant that had arrived as a gift and placed it on Al's chest. "Buddy, I think the plant was in the wrong spot."

Al gave a weak smile and felt the initial embarrassment fade as the raw humor he shared with his old friend fell comfortably over the room. Bob returned with the day shift nurse.

"Did you put that plant on his chest? He is still healing!" The nurse rolled her eyes at Bob Kaye. "I'm so sorry, Mr. Plevier. I should not have let you eat all of your breakfast. You have to slow down."

Quickly, the nurse went about the business of cleaning up her patient and putting the plant back in its proper place.

"Al, I'm still here watching you get a bath." Bob Kaye caught another annoyed look from the nurse and decided to step into the hallway.

Al smiled weakly at his friend. "Thanks, man."

Bob threw another comment over his shoulder as he walked out. "Maybe throwing up helped your lips. You sound better than last week." Bob started to laugh, not allowing Al the opportunity to feel sorry for himself.

"I smell food. Please get rid of it." Al pleaded as another

bout of nausea fell over him.

"Your visitor brought a hamburger for you. I'll toss it in the garbage down the hall." She gently wiped the vomit off Al's face as she reprimanded and simultaneously cajoled him. "One day at a time with your recovery." The gentle woman pulled Al forward to remove his gown and he threw up one more time. "Let's get you changed first and then I'll get myself cleaned up. You shouldn't have food from outside the hospital for the next forty-eight hours."

The nurse cleaned Al, changed his bedding and dressing gown and then let him rest as she carried the dirty linens out of the room. The smell of vomit and stale hamburger hung in the air.

Bob peeked his head into the room. "You decent?"

Al was exhausted. "I'm not gonna be uch company." Bob came in and looked sympathetically at his friend. "You get a sponge bath in this place? Nice."

Al tried to smile. "It's a real spa." Al remembered what he wanted to tell Bob Kaye before he threw up and he rallied from nausea. "Guess who was here? Matt, from the plant."

Bob took a long sip of the coffee he brought with him. "Matt from the Plant? Wasn't he one of the guys who created this mess?"

Al let out a weak, but sarcastic snort. "At first I thought he was here to see how I was."

Bob tried to fill a brief uncomfortable silence. "What was he, the sacrificial lamb for the company?"

Al gave another sarcastic snort. "Guess so. You know what he said? He started off right away with, 'Al the company has rearranged the entire liquid department and made it much safer. Something good came out of this whole mess, right Buddy?' Calls me Buddy, then he says, 'You can't sue the company so I guess management put money into the plant instead of a lawyer.' Matt came all the way down here to tell me almost getting killed, burned and blinded was a good thing." Al continued to vent to his friend. "It blows my mind to think that when I was being interviewed, I asked Mr. Milano about the safety record at the plant." Al stopped

(67)

to catch his breath. "Milano answered me by saying that 'there had been no serious accidents to date'. That should have been my first clue to think twice about taking the job." Al was silent for a several seconds and Bob tried not to cry for his friend. "Know something else? I haven't seen Milano in a week. He used to come by at least every other day and talk to Elaine. I thought he was trying to make up for his behavior on the night I was hurt. Now, nobody calls, nobody comes by."

Bob shook his head and held his hands up to his friend that could not see them. "Look, these guys suck. That's it. You need every ounce of strength you've got to get through this hospital shit. Think about them later." Bob decided instead of making a quick departure, he wouldn't leave the room until he was sure Al fell asleep. "These guys are all business and no balls. You forget about them now and rest. You'll be stronger after you sleep off the vomiting."

Al gave Bob another weak smile and then turned his head toward the ceiling. He tried to focus his mind on the radio, away from his discomfort and drifted fitfully into rest.

After Al had been quiet for a while, Bob was sure he had fallen asleep. He started to leave and ran into Elaine.

Quietly, he spoke to her as he dropped a kiss onto her right cheek. "Our boy here had a rough morning."

Elaine looked over at Al and then back to Bob. "I heard. The day shift nurse met me in the hallway. She asked that we not bring anymore outside food for the next three days except for milkshakes, as long as he doesn't drink three a day."

The nurse, standing behind Elaine, spoke to Bob. "It was nice to meet you." She then turned to Elaine. "I'll be back."

Elaine nodded to the nurse. "Did Al tell you that he's trying to get out of here by Thanksgiving?"

Bob smiled broadly at Elaine. "No, but that's great. I'm sure you can't wait to have him home."

Elaine looked across the room into the air as she thought about caring for her ill and recovering husband. "It will be good to have him home with us. The baby asks for his daddy every day."

Al stirred from the light sleep he was in. "Elaine?"

Elaine stood at the side of his bed. "I'm here, Al. I heard you had a rough morning."

Al yawned and breathed deeply. "I'm exhausted."

Bob looked compassionately at his friend. "I have to get home. Al, I'll be back later this week. Try to keep your food down."

Al smiled weakly. "Thanks, Pal." He heard Bob walk away. "Elaine, I've got to hold my son." Al envisioned his little boy.

"I don't want you to get your hopes up too high because the doctor moved you into this room. He and I were talking about the possibility of Christmas, but Thanksgiving may be an option. Just take it slow." Elaine had to stop as her throat seized.

Torn between the frustration he felt locked in darkness and the understanding of the weight of responsibility placed on the shoulders of his young wife, Al laid in his hospital bed with both fists clenched.

How the hell am I going to do this without becoming a burden to her?

He and Elaine talked most of the afternoon, keeping Al awake until Dr. Westmont made a brief visit late in the day. The doctor informed them that there was a good chance the experimental drug that was used to pull the chemical out of Al's eyes in the emergency room had worked. The testing for Al's ability to see the difference between light and dark proved that a chance existed in the future for a successful corneal transplant. The doctor would not know for sure until the surgery was performed on Al and the doctors could gauge the results.

After Dr. Westmont left the room, Al felt the elation of hope flood through him. He was on a natural high and turned toward his wife. "There's a chance for us to get our life back. We can slip back into our routine and I can take care of my family." Al reached out with his left hand and felt Elaine's.

She wanted to deal with the reality in front of them, but

(69)

instead, she changed the subject. "Al, Dad should be here soon. He said he wanted to talk to the two of us together about something."

"Any idea what he wants to talk about?" Al was still riding high on Dr. Westmont's announcement and did not pick up on Elaine's tension.

"No, but he sounded serious." Elaine released Al's hand and tried to settle into her chair as her father entered the room.

"Afternoon, you two." Mr. Hinds gregarious nature filled a room, even in a hospital.

Al always looked forward to being in his father-in-law's company each day and greeted him warmly. "Hey, Dad."

Mr. Hinds deposited a kiss on Elaine's cheek and stood beside her next to the hospital bed as he spoke to Al. "How you doing today, Boss?"

Al tried to straighten himself in the bed. "Better. Did you hear about this morning?"

"A nurse almost body searched me for food as I came toward the door." Mr. Hinds voice took on a serious tone as he continued. "I ran into Bob in the lobby. He told me you had a visit from Matt."

Al felt the air change in the room and nodded as much as his injuries allowed. "It was the only time I saw him. I haven't heard boo from Milano either in at least a week."

Mr. Hinds dropped his tone and spoke evenly. "We need to talk and now is as good a time as any. You two pay attention to what I'm going to say to you." Mr. Hinds paused for emphasis. "You've been focusing on getting Al well and back home. These visits from guys at the plant are more than goodwill gestures."

Elaine felt the color drain from her face. "Dad, what are you talking about?"

He gave his daughter a sympathetic look. "I knew this was coming. You need a lawyer to look out for you." He turned toward his son-in-law. "Al, you can't work. You're blinded and burned. Do you really think management cares about your family? The company is protecting itself. It's just business." Mr. Hinds looked down at the frightened expression on his daughter's face. He gave the young couple a minute to absorb the information before continuing. "I already talked to Bob Sylvania about this whole mess, and he knows a lawyer through the bank that he wants you both to talk to. You need a tough lawyer to straighten this out and get you back on your feet."

Elaine sighed heavily. "Dad, we're a little overwhelmed. Can't this wait another couple of weeks?"

Looking down into the eyes of his pregnant daughter from his six, foot frame, Mr. Hinds continued. "I get that however, you have no choice. You have to get the ball rolling. This will take months, if not years, to straighten out. There may be statutes of limitations on the time frame allowed for this type of case. You can't get so caught up that it passes by." He turned his attention back to Al. "You're fighting for your family's life, Al. Don't kid yourself. You've always been tougher than most so I know you can handle the battle that started October 1st." Neither Al or Elaine responded. "Look, I'll have Bob Sylvania call the lawyer and have the lawyer call you to make an appointment. You may get busy and push it aside. The lawyer knows how overwhelmed you are right now. He'll call as a favor to Sylvania."

Elaine deferred the arrangements to her father. "Fine, Dad. Do whatever you think is best. We'll follow your lead. Is that all for today?"

Her father nodded. "Yes, but I expect you to take the attorneys calls and cooperate with his directives."

"I promise." She quickly looked to change the subject. "Have you noticed how much Little Albert has grown?"

Mr. Hinds knew what his daughter was doing and went with the flow of the conversation. "Yes, I have. He'll be running bases before we know it." Mr. Hinds was unaware of the impact this line of conversation was having on Al, who lay quietly in his hospital bed.

"I think he's starting to figure out how to get over the gates we've set up." She looked down and patted her stomach. "I wonder if this baby is going to be as active."

Mr. Hinds laughed. "You're going to have double trouble

once the new baby comes and Albert realizes he has competition."

Al formed a mental image of his son the last time he saw him. Little Albert was sitting in his high chair eating breakfast with a huge smile on his face, consistently shoveling cereal pieces, one by one, into his mouth.

"Honestly, I think he grows every time I come home at night to tuck him in. I wonder how he's going to react to the new baby?" She smiled lightly for the first time since her father arrived. "His hair is getting darker now, like your shade, Dad. He's taking after his grandpa's side of the family." Elaine looked over at Al and noticed his stone expression.

"Get out," Al said quietly, almost to himself.

Elaine's expression turned to shock. "What did you say, Al?"

"I said get out." He was about to explode and did not want to unload on the woman he loved most in the world.

"What is it?" Elaine's shock turned to fear.

"I said get out! Both of you, now!" Al thought he might jump out of the bed.

Stunned, the two stared at him before leaving. Al listened to their footfalls and the softly closed door and then let all the emotions of the last three weeks burst out of him as he wept, without tears. He could not remember having cried that hard since he was a four and his mother told him that his daddy was now in heaven.

He felt an intense, overwhelming loss. *Everything is gone. What's the point? How can I help to raise a kid that I can't see? He'll be the only boy on the baseball team with a blind father. How the hell can I ever teach him to throw a ball? Is my father-in-law now going to step in and take over what I can't do? Screw this.*

He was never sure how long the crying jag lasted, but after it subsided, a nurse was at his bedside to offer him some medication. His reply was quick and firm. "No, thank you." Al wasn't sure of all his options, but dulling the emotional pain was not one.

The nurse silently left the room. Al found himself alone in

(72)

the void his imagination had temporarily fooled him into thinking was real. The tearless crying returned, this time harder as his thoughts wandered and images of his own father appeared. He remembered a river where his dad had taken him fishing. In his mind's eye, he could see his dad holding the two poles over his shoulder and a tackle box in his left hand. The conversation between them was simple, short, and comforting, creating a feeling that the world was a safe place. Albert's birth brought back those feelings of innocence and a chance to make up for the life his father was cheated out of. The world was a place that offered second chances to deserving people who worked hard.

He clenched his fists as hard as his injuries allowed. *All my chances are gone. How can a blind man toss a baseball to his son? How can I even help my son with his homework? How can I help Elaine take care of our children? Is she now going to have another kid to take care of? I can't even make a cup of coffee! And the scars. How bad is it, really? Will my son be afraid of me?*

Al, to some degree, would now be dependent on other people. No longer could he drive a car. Someone would always have to be willing to help. The independence that he fought so hard for was slipping through his fingers. At some point, he fell into a fitful sleep. When he awoke, Jack was on duty.

Jack tentatively approached his patient. "How are you doing, Al?"

Al felt a pounding headache. "What time is it?" He felt disoriented.

"Around eight." Jack was told what had happened at the change in shift. He observed Al for signs that the afternoon's meltdown still had a hold on him. "You want me to read to you?"

Al did not want to talk to Jack or anyone else. "Fine." His response was polite but short. He wanted his mind to go blank.

He listened to Jack read from the sportsbook and let his mind wander. Al was happy with the new day shift nurse he was assigned, but Jack stood out as someone who cared about him. The radio he kept on constantly was turned down to a whisper, utilized only for background noise. After a while, Al fell into a sleep of emotional exhaustion that offered no real rest but carried him through the night.

The next day Elaine cautiously entered the hospital room. "Hi Al." She walked over to the bed, wishing she could kiss the lips that were still healing. "How are you?"

Al turned his head toward the only woman he would ever love. "I'm better, babe."

Relief spread over Elaine's face as she looked at her husband. "We'll get through this. We'll make it up as we go along."

Al gave her a nod of acknowledgment and relinquished control of what was lost. "Sell the MG. Let Frank have it for whatever price you think is right. He's been after that car since the day he saw it in our driveway." Al knew letting this friend of the family have the car he loved so dearly would at least bring him closure. "We can use the money."

"You're right." The shock the family experienced almost a month ago had begun to change into acceptance. Knowing Al as she did, she knew that acceptance would become management, as management transitioned them into their new life.

Al smiled. "I'll be home soon. You'll be sick of me in no time."

Chapter VII: The World Beyond

"*At* least my shoes still fit." Al commented to Elaine as he sat on the edge of his hospital bed with his shirt and pants hanging loosely on his thin frame. After six and a half weeks, blind and still recovering physically, he prepared to leave Overlook Hospital and become an outpatient. Relieved to be well enough for discharge, he was anxious about his ability to live at home after being kept in Isolation for the remainder of his recuperation at the hospital. He gripped the rumpled sheets tightly and felt his stomach complain about the earlier skipped breakfast.

He had been eating a diet consisting of normal, bland food to build his strength and determination as he proved to Dr. Euclid and Dr. Westmont that he had the ability to live as an outpatient. Today he questioned the resolve to be home with his family by Thanksgiving knowing the real world outside the walls of the hospital was about to greet him on its own terms. The constant pressure behind his right eye had been building all morning. He was about to mention it to Elaine as a middle-aged social worker came into the room to discuss adapting to the home environment.

At almost six feet tall with thick, bright, red hair, the social worker's presence usually commanded a room the minute she entered, but not for Al. For him, it was the deep resonation of her voice that startled him. "Folks. I've been in touch with the Blind Commission and a representative will be calling you in a day or two." She wasted no time and perfunctorily handed Elaine a manila folder as she continued speaking. "The Blind Commission will be your bridge to other support groups who will continue to help Mr. Plevier and your extended family adjust both socially and physically. Please don't think you can take on the new challenges facing both of you by yourselves or with only the help of your families. You are the ones living with the disability and you need the guidance of someone who is also living with it." She looked from Elaine to Al, trying to gauge their comprehension of the adjustment ahead of them. "You can still call me with any questions on available resources. This is a lifetime commitment to your new family circumstances."

Feeling panic begin to rise inside of him, Al decided to be flip and hopefully end the lecture. "I'm ready for a change, but I think I might need a new wardrobe." He pulled at his shirt for effect.

The social worker looked strangely at him and then continued. "You have lost quite a bit of weight. I'm sure being home will help you put the weight back on."

This lady is dry. "I guess. But I'd be more comfortable naked.*"*

Elaine stepped between the social worker and Al. "Thank you for all your help. Al, let's get started. I still have some papers to sign."

His weight had plummeted from 165 pounds before the accident to 130 pounds at his lowest during the hospital stay. Today it stood at 138 pounds and Al had fought hard to gain those eight pounds back. In Overlook, he had worn only a hospital gown after he was moved to Isolation. Today he sat on the edge of his bed wearing blue jeans and a white T-shirt that no longer fit, a reminder of a life that no longer existed.

Will I fit anywhere now?

His fear and apprehension about joining the outside world began to build and he tried to think of something else. "What's the weather like outside?" Al asked tilting his head toward Elaine.

The social worker looked up from writing on her notepad not realizing Al had directed the question to his wife. "The weather is a bit chilly." She then turned to Elaine. "Did you bring a coat for him?"

"Yes. Al, I laid it next to you on the pillow." She turned to try and coax the social worker out of the room. "I think we're almost ready to go. Do you need me to sign off for your visit with us?" Elaine looked at the notepad and clipboard the woman held.

"Yes, please," the busy woman commented with a smile, glad to be moving on with her day.

Al had listened to the conversation between the two women and felt invisible. He was aware why Elaine did not ask if he needed to sign the paperwork. *I can't sign my name anymore. How the hell am I going to move forward? I won't be able to do anything without my wife.* The pressure behind his eye grew with his internal monologue. *The world won't adjust for me. I don't expect it to.*

Elaine looked over her shoulder at Al. "Honey, I'll be right back with an orderly. Hospital policy requires that you are released in a wheelchair."

The empty space the exiting women left in the room intensified the quiet. *Home. Home is Where the Heart Is and my heart wants to hide in this bed. What was I thinking to insist I be out of here by Thanksgiving? I'm not ready and my head is killing me.* Al began wringing his hands together, tearing his new skin, and immediately regretted it. *Maybe home ain't looking so good right now. How can I help manage our life together? I can't even look someone in the eye. I'll have to constantly listen to the changes in their voices to distinguish truth from lies.* Al bent his head down and tried to quell the fear washing over him. *Man, I'm on my own. My wife can't stop life from happening to me.*

Elaine came back into the room with a tall, thin, man pushing the promised wheelchair. "Come on, Hon. It's time to go home." Elaine stepped aside to let the orderly push the wheelchair in front of Al.

Al raised his head slightly, "Home." He tried not to sound

sarcastic or as scared as he felt. He reached for his coat and found it next to him as Elaine had promised. Carefully, he slipped his arms into the light jacket. "How faraway did you park?"

Elaine tried to maintain a positive disposition in spite of the ache that had begun in her lower back. "Not far, but I will pull the car to the front door." Not realizing that Al's anxiety originated from the car ride ahead, Elaine furrowed her brow and wondered if every bit of minutia was going to become a major obstacle. "The orderly will wait with you."

Al eased himself off the bed and felt the hand of the orderly on his left upper arm guiding him to the wheelchair. He tapped the man's hand to let him know he was capable of getting into the chair himself. He stood next to his bed and reached into the air in front of him and down until his hands collided with the arms of the wheelchair. Slowly he turned himself around and lowered his body into the familiar seat.

The orderly held the chair firmly. "Let's get you downstairs. I know you're anxious to get home." He smiled at Elaine.

Al sat with his head down and hoped Elaine remembered that he wanted a quiet homecoming. "Who's at the house?"

"Just Ronnie, as we planned. She will probably leave after you're settled in." She picked up the black bag containing Al's few possessions. "I want to stop by and give the nurses the gifts I bought for them so I will meet you at the front door with the car. Take your time coming down." The discomfort in her lower back increased slightly and Elaine tried to hurry from the room. She was stopped short at the door by more nervous conversation from Al as he called after her.

"Maybe I should have waited another couple of weeks." Al let his thoughts slip out and he was immediately sorry.

"It's going to be okay, Al." Elaine knew her husband needed reassurance because she needed it so badly herself. "Take a breath and relax." Elaine tried to calm the anxiety she had been Feeling about what lay ahead of her with her own internal dialogue. *I can do this. First things first. Let's get him home. I want us all*

(78)

together, like it should be. My family will be together under one roof tonight. I'll call my Obstetrician after I get Al settled in. The back ache is probably due to all the tension today. We're going to be fine. My family will be together tonight. Elaine walked out of the room without giving Al another chance to stop her.

He heard her footfalls moving away and fell silent as the orderly slowly backed the chair up. *What do I look like? People in the real world won't understand. I must look like shit.*

He had always been a clean, shaven man, but on this day, a week before Thanksgiving, he resembled Van Gogh. Blond since birth, his hair had turned to brown and was constantly oily even after shampooing. The decrease in facial swelling within weeks after the chemical onslaught required him to cope with the baby soft skin with miraculous facial hair that could not be shaved.

The gentle orderly heard Al take a deep breath. "The worst is over, Mr. Plevier. Anybody that can live through your ordeal is a survivor."

Al lifted his head, "Thanks, Buddy." *I can do this. I feel myself getting better. It's slow, but I feel it. Life goes on.*

"Mr. Plevier do you want to say goodbye to anyone?" The orderly could see the tension on Al's face.

Al really wanted to slip out a side door into a different reality. "Tell me, how bad do I really look?"

The orderly looked Al over thoughtfully. "You have this unshaven, un-shampooed thing going on, but with the bandages and goggles on your eyes, I think people will forgive you. Those things look like unfashionable eye glasses from the fifties with their heavy aluminum sides and large lenses. The removable bandages give people the clue that you have a medical need for them and not that you have bad taste."

Al laughed lightly at the bold honesty. "I guess that's better than the alternative." He tried to straighten up, but lifting his head exaggerated the constant drumming behind his eye.

The orderly looked Al over to see if he was ready to move. "What do you think? Are you ready to roll?"

Al had grown accustomed to wheelchair and elevator rides

(79)

within the confines of Overlook, but the dread of the approaching car ride scared him. "Not really." He let his hands grip the chair arms and turned his head toward the orderly. "What's your name?"

The patient man held the handles of the wheelchair. "Henry."

"You sound to be about six feet tall, Henry. Am I right?"

"Close, Mr. Plevier." Henry looked down at the injured man.

Al took one last deep breath and released it slowly. "Let's do this." The orderly pulled Al backward out of the small room. "You'll be happy to be home and have some of your wife's cooking, I'm sure."

Al laughed. "You got that right. Anything, even Elaine's cooking, is better than what the hospital feeds me."

The orderly whistled low as he pulled Al into the hallway and began to push him forward. "You better keep that to yourself."

Someone walking by stopped them. "So, it's moving day, huh, Mr. Plevier? Good for you. Congratulations."

"Who's that?" Al didn't recognize the voice but knew it was familiar.

"It's Danny, from therapy." The young man reached out and touched Al's left shoulder. "We're going to miss you around here. Take care of yourself."

Recognition spread across Al's face. "Oh, sorry. I didn't catch who you were."

Danny smiled down at his former patient. "Don't worry about it. I think you're a little preoccupied on your big day. I'm glad to see you're on your way home." Danny took his hand away and nodded in the direction of the orderly. "Safe trip home, Mr. Plevier."

"Thanks for everything. You were wonderful to me." Al felt the wheelchair push forward.

As the wheelchair passed the nurses' station several women called out to him. The first voice Al recognized was the woman that saved him from Mary. "Take care, Mr. Plevier."

The second voice could have been a new nurse. "It's good

to see you leaving. We'll miss you."

Al did not ask the orderly to stop but simply called back to the kind women. "Thanks ladies, for everything. You were wonderful to me and my family. I'll never forget any of you."

After traveling a short distance, the wheelchair came to a stop and Al heard the familiar ding of the elevator. He was pulled backward into the metal box and as it began its descent, he felt his stomach tighten. "Here we go."

The kind man looked over Al's shoulder. "How are you doing?"

Al brushed off his worries. "Fine. I won't throw up, I promise."

The doors opened upon the first, floor landing and he felt the change of air as a cool draft played across his face and hands. Subconsciously he gripped the arms of the wheelchair and clenched his jaw.

I'm not ready for the car. No way.

"We're heading for the front door. If your wife isn't there yet, we can wait in the lobby." The wheelchair continued straight and then came to a stop as another substantial drop in temperature assaulted his body.

We must be at the front door. The air is so cold. It feels awful on my skin. Why didn't someone give me a blanket to wrap around my shoulders? It's so cold. I can't do this. I need to stay here a little while longer until I can garner more strength. The car ride will make me sick. Elaine was never a great driver. She hates driving. There are so many trucks up this way. How is she going to handle having me in the car? I guess she had lots of practice with the trucks these last six weeks. I don't want to do this. I can't do this.

"You're awfully quiet." The orderly looked down at Al's head.

"I'm fine," Al mumbled almost incoherently.

"Your wife should be here any second." The orderly pushed the chair forward through the outer doors and the outside air smacked Al's healing skin like a wet towel.

(81)

Al pulled his coat closer and then felt more than heard a car pull up in front of him. Instinctively, he recoiled. A car door opened and slammed shut. He heard someone walk quickly to his side.

Elaine stood between Al and the car door. "Let's go home." She opened the passenger side door of the Oldsmobile station wagon. "You're right in front of the curb, so when you get out of the chair, step down.

Al let Elaine guide him as he tentatively felt for the curb with his foot. With his right hand, he felt for the car door and slid into the passenger seat instinctively ducking his head under the frame. He felt the seat give way under his weight as he slipped, uncomfortably, into his new place in life.

I guess this is Elaine's car now. I will never have a sense of freedom driving. A wave of intense sadness washed over him as he breathed in deeply. *This is going to be a long drive.* Al wriggled in the seat, letting the physicality of the car remove him temporarily from the confines of his emotions. *I never realized how much these seats force you forward at the waist. Maybe I should have lain down in the back seat. I feel like I'm going to go through the windshield.*

Elaine ducked down until her head was next to Al's. "Hon for today, would you mind wearing your seat belt? It would make me feel better." Elaine did not give Al time to make a choice, instead pulled the belt across his waist and clicked it into place.

Buckling me in like a child. Is she kidding? "Just for the ride home, but I have to tell you, this thing is killing me already." The irony of the fact that before the accident he never wore a seat belt in any car was not lost on him. *What the hell am I being careful for now? I'm already blind and scarred. How much more can be done to me?*

Elaine was not feeling well and decided to ignore his comment. "You're buckled in. Let's go." She slammed the door shut and started to walk around the car, waving to the orderly. "Thank you for all your help."

"Goodbye, folks." The nice man pulled the chair back.

(82)

Elaine climbed into the driver's side, tucking her growing stomach behind the wheel and then buckled her own seat belt. "Here we go, Al. Our family is together."

Here we go. Al barely heard Elaine put the car into drive as it pulled away from the curb. He grabbed the arm rest and almost opened the door accidentally. *I feel like I'm on an amusement park ride. Did she always drive this erratically?*

"Elaine, can you give me a little warning before you start or stop?" Al knew he sounded snotty.

"We haven't left the parking lot. Try to relax. You'll get used to the motion of the car." Elaine hoped she conveyed her weary tone.

The car made a right turn, sped up and then reached a steady speed. *I'm going to be sick. I need air. How am I supposed to take this for an hour?* "Elaine, can you pull over?"

"You'll have to wait until I find a safe place. Try to relax. Why don't you roll down the window as much as you can? If the air doesn't help and you still feel nauseous, we'll pull over." Elaine gripped the steering wheel.

Al tried to counter his anxiety with continuous conversation. "How's traffic?" He knew Elaine was getting annoyed but did not care.

Elaine stared straight while replying. "Not bad. We're moving along. Can you tell that our speed has increased?"

Just then a truck barreled past the station wagon blaring its horn and shook the car from the wind tunnel it had created. Al now had his left hand dug so deeply into the seat he knew the upholstery would never be the same.

He cringed inwardly and worked out a solution for his anxiety. *Next car ride I'm asking for medication. I can't handle this. Was she always such a lousy driver? She should drive slower. I've got to put the window down and hang my head out. With any luck, I'll fall out.* He started to push down the window button with his injured right arm and when it was a third of the way opened, he leaned toward the fresh air. The blast of cold eased his nausea.

"Al, what are you doing? Don't lean so far, you're going to hurt yourself." Elaine hated to admit it, but she wondered if the doctor had released him before he was truly ready.

Al pulled himself back to sitting straight and felt his injuries respond accordingly. "I need air, but it's worse now. With the window down everything is louder." He knew there was nothing that could be done to alleviate his fears or nausea. "Elaine, you drive too fast. We'll have to find somebody else to drive us."

"Relax. I'm not driving fast I'm driving at the speed limit." Elaine took a breath and tried to control her own anxieties and alleviate a persistent backache that only seemed to increase. "No one is going to drive us around. I'll get used to doing all the driving and so will you." She gripped the steering wheel tightly.

Al breathed out deeply and dug his nails further into the seat. "Where are we? Are we close to home?"

"We've only been on the road for ten minutes. Please, relax. I have to concentrate on driving."   Elaine stared at the road and the traffic ahead of her. "Really, the traffic is not bad this time of the morning. We missed rush hour."

"Just get me home and cement my butt to the sofa, that's all I ask." Al took a deep breath but it did nothing to alleviate the tense feeling in his chest and the constantly building pressure behind his right eye.

"Why don't we talk about Little Albert?" Elaine was trying desperately to ignore her growing discomfort.

He breathed out deeply and loosened his grip on the seat. "I can't wait to be near him." Al voiced a fear he tried to keep from Elaine. "Do you think he'll be afraid of me?" He turned his head toward the passenger side window. "What about the eye bandages and the protective covers? He might try to pull them off."

Elaine smiled for the first time during the drive. Your fast progress is amazing. Your face is red but you look like yourself, except for the eye bandages and goggles." She hoped this vote of confidence would ease his concern about how Albert would react to seeing his father. "I think the baby will be more curious about your goggles than anything else." She felt her stomach cramp slightly, ran her hand over it and wished the trip would end so that she could lie down. She thought about the relief of stretching out on her own bed as another cramp started. Suddenly she knew this was more than stress. She had to get her husband home quickly and then take care of herself. "Don't worry about the glasses. We'll keep his hands away. He'll learn quickly not to touch Daddy's eyes."

Al lifted his head to face the windshield and tried to forget the feelings of self-pity that were beginning to resurface. "We'll have fun together, he and I. Right now, I just want to hold him." Al remembered the last time he saw Albert sitting at the table in his high chair. Al had stopped before heading toward the back door, his coffee mug in his hand and kissed the baby on the top of his head.

"Al? Where are you?" Elaine thought she would enjoy the silence, but the quiet amplified her cramping.

He turned his head toward her as the tires of the passing cars reacted to the paved roadway. "I'm with you, Sweetheart, going home." The discomfort from his healing body started to regain its momentum and he shifted nervously in his seat.

"Are you in pain?" Elaine thought about her own intensifying backache and understood how the car ride must feel to her husband.

Al shifted and rubbed his back against the seat. "Can you give me updates on how close we are?"

"Sure. We've been on the road about fifteen minutes." Elaine stayed in the right lane and let traffic fly by her at what seemed like dizzying speeds to Al. "I'm doing the speed limit, so don't get your hopes up for a quick arrival."

"No problem." Al renewed his death grip on the seat and armrest. "I feel like we're on a ride at an amusement park. The cars and trucks are so loud."

Elaine glanced over at her husband. "Can you tell the difference between cars and trucks?"

"Are you kidding?" He shook his head slowly. "It's like

(85)

the trucks are dragging us with them."

Elaine closed her eyes and quickly opened them. She worked to have the necessary patience for this car ride and all the rides ahead for her family. "I guess you're getting inundated with all sensations you never noticed before."

Al interrupted her with irritation. "It's the unknown. It's the fear of what I can't see. If I could see it, I'd understand it. Now I have to have it explained to me. I know a truck is a truck and not a car, but to me, each one is barely missing our car. Everything is so loud. I feel like I'm sitting with my head between two speakers turned up to ten."

Elaine gripped the wheel tighter and felt sweat form in her palms. "We're safe. Don't expect to process all of this today. You're still healing."

Al's irritation grew. "Let me know how close we are to our exit." The multitude of noises continued to assault Al for the duration of the journey home. Sitting still he attempted to put his mind somewhere else. *I don't know what is worse, the outside noises I'm trying to identify or trying to explain to Elaine what is going on inside my head. This is exhausting. She's slowing down. This has to be the exit. She's coming to a stop. Are we in the driveway?* Automatically Al reached for the door handle.

"Al! What are you doing? We're at the off ramp on the highway!" Elaine panicked and her body responded accordingly.

"Whoa! Sorry. I thought we were home." He jerked back away from the door.

Elaine breathed out deeply. "We're almost home. Another five minutes. We're on Riverview Drive." *Please, God. Let me get him home safely, and then I will get myself to the hospital.*

In his mind's eye, Al saw the picturesque street as it had been on October first with the leaves beginning their fiery exit. He knew now it must be leafless during this in between time of seasons. He felt the car slow and make another turn.

"Al, we're pulling into the driveway," Elaine felt like shouting from the rooftops for more than one reason. "Welcome home, Sweetheart."

Without thinking twice, Al reached to unbuckle the seatbelt that had held him captive, opened the door and felt cold air slap at his body for a third time today. He turned in the seat, let his feet touch the ground as he stood, feeling the gravel under his shoes.

Elaine unbuckled herself and gingerly climbed out from behind the steering wheel. The cramping was reaching a crescendo and, in her heart, she knew what it meant. Still keeping her presence of mind, she looked at her husband over the roof of the car and then retrieved the cane the hospital had given them.

Ronnie walked over carrying Little Albert. "Welcome home, Al." Little Albert screeched and waved his hands.

Al walked around the front of the car, running his hand along the hood for guidance. "Hey, little guy! How you doing?"

Elaine watched Al's progress as her need to get into the house grew. "Al, we're directly in front of the back door. You're facing the forsythia bush that's by the kitchen window."

He continued toward the sound of Elaine's voice and then felt her place the cane in his left hand. "Thanks."

"It will help you get used to navigating around the house." A strong cramp began to build as Elaine struggled to focus on Al.

Immediately Al became defensive at the limits now imposed upon him. "I can count my steps. I don't need this thing around here."

Elaine held her hand over his left hand. "I know how you feel about this, but it will help initially until you count the steps and remember where the obstacles are in the house and yard." Elaine was breathing deeply both for patience and the growing pain in her lower back. "Put your right hand on my shoulder. Use me and the cane. Slow. Perseverance. Remember?"

Al and Elaine made their way directly toward the back door and he felt the gravel beneath his shoes crunch with familiarity. "It still smells like fall but it feels like winter." He resisted the urge to reach down and let the gravel run through his fingers.

"The river is coming up a little high. We've had a lot of rain this week." Elaine tried to move slowly for Al, but she longed to get inside as the cramping grew in intensity. "Al, you're at the

(87)

steps. Ronnie is at the top. I have to get inside."

Al squeezed Elaine's shoulder and then let it go. "I got it, one step at a time."

Ronnie watched her sister closely and opened her mouth to say something but was silenced by the sight of Elaine's pale face. "Al, what do you need me to do?"

Al had tucked the cane under his left arm and started to climb the six steps. "Stay out of the way."

Ronnie smiled. "Got it. The baby wants you."

Albert actually wanted to follow his mother but as Ronnie kept a tight hold on him, he turned his attention to his dad. He pointed to Al and then opened and closed his little fist with an accompanying greeting. "Hi."

Al carefully climbed each step, not wanting to fall down on his face and create more drama for his wife. He reached the top step, felt for the door frame in front of him, and turned his head toward the little voice he had heard. "Hi to you too. Remember me?" The smells of coffee, baby and life drifted into his senses. He breathed in deeply. "Home."

Ronnie spoke around the lump in her throat. "Yes, you're home and this little guy is very happy about that." She moved to the side as Al began to shuffle through the doorway. "Let me shut that door so Little Al doesn't make a run for it."

Al moved farther into the kitchen, still refusing to use his cane. "Thanks." He tried by memory to find his way to the end of the breakfast counter as Ronnie closed the back door. His feet shuffled as he tried to step. Gravel from the driveway scratched the lime and gold linoleum floor until he reached the edge of the counter where he promptly hung the cane.

I'm alive. I made it back. My son is only a few feet away from me. "Is anyone interested in lunch?" In reality, he had no interest in food, but spoke in the direction he thought Ronnie and the baby were in not realizing, they had already walked to the other side of the room.

Ronnie put the active toddler on his feet and he ran toward his father. "That sounds great, Al. I think the baby could eat more bananas and I'm always ready for more food."

Al shot his head around to where Ronnie stood and immediately regretted the effect the movement had on the pounding behind his right eye. He tried to cover his disorientation. "I would love something hot, like tea. I don't drink coffee now."

Ronnie watched the little boy stand next to his father and stare up at him. "I'll get right to it. Al, the baby is on your left."

Still holding on to the counter Al felt the need to sit down as he felt toward his left and lightly tapped Albert's head. "I'm going into the family room." He heard Albert run away, yelling joyfully into his toy area ahead. "Where did Elaine go?"

Ronnie thought back to her sister's pale face and thought she might have needed to lie down in the bedroom. "I don't know. Maybe she had to use the bathroom. It's a long drive."

She saw her brother-in-law tentatively moving toward the family room and realized the obstacle course Albert's toys would make. "Do you want me to help you navigate?"

Al tried not to be defensive but could not contain his anger at being treated like he had a handicap. "I'm home because I can handle it. You don't have to hover."

Ronnie rolled her eyes as she took out a plate and a mug. "Take the cane. Albert's toys are everywhere."

Out of stubbornness and desperation to maintain some semblance of normalcy, Al had left the cane hooked over the counter and felt his way to the family room entrance. He shuffled to the right as he tried to gauge where the sofa was in reference to the doorway. He kicked objects out of his way before he stubbed his foot on something firm and realized it might be the edge of the red sofa. Bending over slightly, he ran his hand along the familiar material of the sofa arm encountering two more of Little Al's toys and then Albert.

"Whatcha doing, Buddy?" Al turned and sat down with the ease, familiarity and relief of being home.

"Hi." Little Al opened and closed his fist in front of his dad.

"Hi to you too, Albert." Al smiled for his son and tried to

ignore his headache.

Ronnie came into the family room with the cane hooked over her wrist. "I'm still making you a sandwich but here are some tea and cookies to hold you over. Where should I put them?" Al thought about the baby toddling in front of him and wondered the same thing. "I guess give me the tea and I'll hang on to it so Albert doesn't grab for it. He and I will share the cookies."

As soon as Ronnie put the plate down on the coffee table in front of the sofa, the toddler went for a cookie. "Better get one soon or there won't be any left." Ronnie carefully placed the tea handle in front of Al's right hand and touched it to his fingers.

He slipped his fingers through the handle. "Thanks."

She started back to the kitchen, calling over her shoulder. "I put the cane next to you, in case."

"In case what? Afraid I'm going to take a header over a toy?" The headache continued to build.

"Another minute of listening to you snipe at me and I think I'll just let you do that. You haven't been home ten minutes and you're already cranky." Ronnie smiled, glad to see the fight in her brother-in-law. "After you finish your tea, why don't you go find your wife." Ronnie looked over at Al and for the first time since the accident, she felt that her sister's family would do more than survive the horror. "Good luck navigating the toys."

"You're a real sweetheart." Al felt next to the sofa where he had heard Ronnie place the cane and grasped it in his left hand. "Thanks." He sat in the family room for a half hour, speaking quietly to his son and trying to imagine how the baby looked toddling around the room in front of him. He gave a silent thank you to Ronnie for not making conversation with him as he sat drinking his warm tea and battling the growing headache and the constant burn discomfort.

He finished his tea and then clumsily placed it on the table in front of him. Slowly rising from the couch, he stopped short, reached down, and gripped the cane. Moving forward, he navigated around both his son and scattered toddler paraphernalia as he started toward the master bedroom to look for Elaine.

"Albert, Daddy is going to look for Mommy." Al felt his foot stub something light and he quickly brushed it aside.

Albert looked up from the coffee table where he had proudly brought his blocks, one by one, in front of his dad. "Mama."

Al smiled at Albert's voice and continued to move around the table and toward the bedroom hallway. "Yes, Mama. You stay here and keep Aunt Ronnie company." Al yelled to Ronnie over his shoulder and immediately felt the reverberation inside his head. "Ron? I'm going to look for Elaine."

Ronnie looked up from the sandwich she was making. "Go ahead. I've got a handle on the little guy." She walked toward Albert and prepared to sit down and play with him. "We're great pals, he and I."

Each movement of the cane shifted the pressure behind Al's right eye like the water in a fish tank shifted by an earthquake. He kept moving carefully across the family room until he found the entrance to the hallway exactly where he expected it to be. The combination of a headache and the discomfort from the healing burns played on his ability to remember and memorize the foot print of the home. He thought he had found the doorway leading to the master bedroom, turned right and walked into the half open linen closet door.

"Dammit!" Al exclaimed aloud and then was instantly sorry. He felt along the wall until he knew he was at the next doorway. Utilizing the cane, he cautiously entered and quietly spoke to his wife. "Elaine?" After not getting an immediate response, he tried again. "Elaine? Are you all right?"

He heard Elaine's voice coming from the master bathroom. "I'm in here, Al. I don't feel well."

Al shuffled toward the bathroom and swung the cane to his right trying to find the end of the bed. He sat down heavily and waited for Elaine.

The door opened with its familiar creak and she walked toward her husband. "Something is wrong. I need to go to the hospital right now." Elaine could no longer hide the pain.

(91)

Al froze and forgot about his own pain. "Oh my God. Let's call your mother or somebody to go with you."

Elaine shook her head as tears flowed down her cheeks. "There's no time. I'll get myself to Wayne Paterson General. I'll have Ronnie call Mom and Dad to tell one of them to meet me." Elaine stopped as another pain washed over her.

"Wait!" Al felt panic begin to set in. "Please, you can't drive like that." He started to stand.

Elaine turned to leave the room. "Al, I have to go. Call Ronnie if you need something."

Al yelled to the empty air in front of him. "Elaine!" He knew his wife had left and sat on the edge of the bed before moving to the doorway. He listened for activity and heard Ronnie talking to Albert. "Ronnie?"

Ronnie came across the living room and into the hallway entrance. "Al?"

"I'm fine. Where is Elaine?" Al gripped the door frame tightly as the pressure behind his eye grew into a thrumming that would not cease.

Ronnie looked down at the carpet and tried not to cry. "Al, she left. She couldn't wait for anyone."

Silence fell over them until Albert pushed his aunt to move her out of his way. "Dada."

Al slowly knelt down to his son's level and winced at the accompanying vibration in his head. "How about if you hang out with Aunt Ronnie. Dada is going to take his medicine and lie down."

Ronnie tried to coax the little boy back to her. "Come on kiddo, let's play trucks." At the sound of the word trucks, the toddler ran back to the family room. "Al, Elaine didn't have time to tell me what to do with your medicine. Do you know which one you need now?"

Al tried to think coherently around what had become a blinding headache. "Not really. Elaine has a notebook that she writes everything down in. Did you call your parents?"

"Yes, before Elaine was out the door. Mom will meet her

at the hospital and Dad is trying to get off early so he can stay with you." Ronnie looked over her shoulder at Albert. "Will you be able to wait for your medication until Dad gets here?"

He thought about how wonderful Ronnie was with Albert. "I'll be fine. As soon as he gets here we'll get on track with my medications. The pressure behind my eye is getting worse so I need to lie down. Dad will give me the codeine later."

Ronnie sat next to Albert on the floor. "I'm going to call Dad at work and rush him. I'll keep the baby out of your room."

Al turned around and made his way to the queen size bed he shared with Elaine. Unable to see, he welcomed the familiar feel of the mattress as he lowered his body onto the edge, slowly swung his legs up and tried to lie down against the pillows. His head screamed with pain as he leaned back.

Elaine, I'm so sorry I'm not with you.

He removed the safety goggles given to him at the hospital and placed them on the nightstand. He stayed in that position and tried to relax and calm the pain that was building behind his eyes until he heard his father-in-law call his name.

"Al? How you doing, Son?" Mr. Hinds came into the master bedroom carrying a small plastic pill bottle and a glass of water.

"Hi, Dad." Al didn't bother to try to lift his throbbing head off the pillows. "How is Elaine?"

Mr. Hinds came to the side of the bed and tried to speak as low as possible. "I don't know yet. We're waiting for your mother-in-law to call. I have a glass of water and your codeine." He let the glass touch Al's left hand.

Al grasped it gratefully. "Thanks, Dad."

"I'm putting two of the pills in your right hand." He looked at his son- in-law and wondered if the doctors and Elaine had both been too eager to have Al home before Thanksgiving.

Al threw the codeine pills to the back of his throat and swallowed. He knew he only had a few moments before he would be overtaken by the narcotic's effects. "Please, try to wake me if you hear something from the hospital."

"I will." He looked at Al, still in his jeans and t-shirt. "Do you need help getting out of your pants?"

Al realized getting them off was probably a good idea but dreaded the effects on his headache. "Nah, I got it. Just give me a little privacy."

"Call me if you need anything." Mr. Hinds left.

Al sat up on the edge of the bed and tried to wiggle out of the jeans. Immediately the pills began to take effect. He unsnapped his pants in his seated position and then slipped them over his hips pushing them past the baby soft new skin on his legs. Clothed in his boxers and the white t-shirt, he allowed the pain medication to work.

Chapter VIII: Reconciliation

Al awoke at around one o'clock in the morning, confused and groggy. At first, he thought he was at Overlook. "Jack, what time is it?" When he didn't receive an answer, he reached for the hospital call button always strapped to the side of his bedrail. "Jack?"

The sound of footsteps, much softer than usual, came into his room. "Son? Try not to yell if you can help it. You might wake the little guy." Mr. Hinds walked into the bedroom, coming to a stop next to Al's side of the bed.

Al stayed in the confused state, thinking he was at Overlook and his father-in-law had come for a visit, but he knew the "Little Guy" would not be with him. His mind began to clear and then spoke into the silence.

"Dad, where's Elaine?" Before another thought could enter Al's mind, the ache behind his right eye began to drum.

Mr. Hinds swallowed hard. "Son, she's at the hospital. Remember, yesterday?"

Suddenly, Al was fully awake. "Yesterday?"

Mr. Hinds realized the confused state his son was in. "It's after midnight. The drugs the doctors gave you knocked you out.

You've been asleep for twelve hours." Mr. Hinds looked more closely at his son-in-law and wondered if he should either take him to the emergency room or wake up one of his doctors.

Silence enveloped the two men as the events of yesterday came rushing back to Al. "Dad, how is Elaine?"

The older man looked sadly at his son-in-law. "Mom called after dinner. Elaine is resting comfortably and will be staying overnight at the hospital." Mr. Hinds swallowed hard. "Al, I'm sorry, she lost the baby."

Al remained still until he reached to the nightstand and knocked over a glass of water. He let his hand lie on the table top. "This is all my fault."

The room fell silent. The tick tock of the battery-operated alarm clock Elaine refused to part with rattled the ominous air until Mr. Hinds broke the silence. "Son, you're alive. This baby was not meant to be. Imagine what today would be like if she did not have you to come home to."

The vision of Elaine standing next to a grave had never crossed his mind even during the ambulance ride to Overlook. That afternoon he acted on instinct begging for death to get relief. If he had not lived, tomorrow she would have asked whoever drove her home from the hospital to stop by the graveyard. Through tears she would have clutched her arms weakly around herself, burying her chin as far into her chest as it would allow. Shaking her head slowly from side to side she would have tried to make sense of the massacre to her young family. She would have cried over how life can change in an instant from one of hope to one of finding the strength to move beyond repetitive grief. Instead, tomorrow, Al would be there to comfort her and offer the hope that their family could still grow. The two of them could have more children. Elaine would need him now and he would take care of *her*.

"Dad?" Al struggled to think beyond the pain behind his right eye.

Mr. Hinds could see the strain in his face. "Yes?"

"Thanks for helping us. We would be lost without all of you." Al breathed heavily.

(96)

Mr. Hinds continued what he had started by walking silently to the bathroom to retrieve a hand towel and wipe up the water Al had knocked over. "You want another pill?"

Al ran his right hand along the comforter in the empty space next to him. "Yes, please." Al remembered other medication he was sent home with. "Dad, I need the drop for my eyes. It might help with the pain."

The older man went to the kitchen and brought back the small pharmacy Al was sent home with. "I'm going to keep these on top of the fridge for now. Elaine can do what she wants with them tomorrow."

"She's coming home definitely tomorrow?" Al felt Mr. Hinds put a pill in his hand and heard another glass placed on the oak night stand.

"Yes. Tomorrow afternoon is what Mom told me on the phone. The doctor wanted to keep her overnight so she could rest." Mr. Hinds groped through the bag of medicine until he found the drop bottle. "How do you want to do this? Should I put the drops in?"

Al reached carefully for the glass of water as he spoke. "No, I don't want you to feel uncomfortable. I can do it as long as I have someone standing by to direct me." He threw the pill in his hand into his mouth and washed it down. "Dad, can you give me the drop bottle?" Al felt the bottle placed in his hand and put down the glass he still held in the other hand. He lifted the bandages covering his right eye, tipped his head back and immediately felt the pressure and pain already there build further. "Dad, you have to let me know if some drops come out. I only need three or four." Al brought the drop bottle to the edge of his right eye and prepared to let the medication enter.

"Maybe I should do that." Mr. Hinds began to reach for the drop bottle as he watched Al squeeze three or four drops from the bottle. "That's enough. Stop."

Al moved the bottle away from his eye and began to feel the effects of the codeine ease his headache. "You're about to lose me, Dad. Take the bottle." Al quickly replaced the bandages.

(97)

"I'll check on you throughout the night. If you need me, call out, I'm sleeping in the guest bedroom." He watched Al's head go heavy on the pillow barricade surrounding his upper body. Mr. Hinds walked across the hall to the nursery to check on the baby and then found his way to the guest bedroom. Exhausted and emotionally drained, he collapsed onto the bed fully dressed and without the comfort of covers.

In the morning, the first person to awaken was Little Albert. "Mamamama?"

His grandpa opened his eyes slowly and looked at the bright morning sun outlining the privacy shade on the east facing window. As the toddler called out, Elaine's father stretched and slowly raised himself off of the bed. "I'm coming little guy."

Realizing this was not his mother's voice, the toddler began to cry until he reached a crescendo that woke Al. The hangover effects of the one codeine pill and his throbbing head cemented him to the bed. He had no idea what time it was, but he knew by the way he felt that he could have only been asleep for four or five hours. The events of yesterday came rushing back to him and Elaine's face was framed in his mind. He fought his way through the residual medication and began to carefully shift his body.

I wish I could be of some help to Dad.

The baby's screams subsided a bit in the other room as Albert raised his arms to the familiar face of his grandfather. "Grandpa's here. Let's get a fresh diaper on you, and we'll both have breakfast." The older man lifted his grandson out of the crib and yawned loudly. "Your grandpa needs coffee."

As his grandfather carried him out of the nursery, Albert pointed to the master bedroom. "Dada."

"Very good, you remembered your dad came home yesterday. You want to go see your pop this morning?" Mr. Hinds peeked into the bedroom and found Al adjusting his upper body carefully on the bed. Softly he called to him. "Hey."

Al lifted his head toward the voice. "Morning, Dad. I heard the baby fussing to get up. Sorry I can't help out yet."

Little Albert was in fourth gear the second his eyes opened

and now the energetic toddler fought to get out of his grandfather's arms and climb into Al's. "You just take care of yourself, Son." Mr. Hinds released Albert and watched him run toward the living room. "Al, I have to keep an eye on the baby, but if you feel up to it, come into the kitchen and I'll get you something to eat."

Al, still in the same T-shirt he wore yesterday, tried to sit forward off the support of the pillows surrounding him and hold his head upright. The drumming behind his eye intensified.

He fought the growing pain by holding onto his last image of his wife from the morning of October 1. "Give me a couple minutes to get myself going, Dad. I'll be out as soon as I can."

Mr. Hinds watched Al's face closely. "If you need medication before Elaine comes home let me know, but you have to get food into you first."

"You take care of the baby. I'll be out soon." He continued to hang onto the image of Elaine looking over her shoulder at him as she tossed her hair.

Al listened to the sound of his father-in-law's movement away from the bedroom and then began to slowly lift his head and shoulders from the small comfort the pillows gave him. He brought his knees toward his chest as he tried to steady himself. The reverberation in his head was extreme after he swung his legs over to and his feet touched the carpet.

He lost his image of Elaine while, ten miles away, she prepared to be driven home by her mother after the overnight stay at Wayne General Hospital. Elaine was stoic as she was wheeled out of the hospital, but she burst into tears as soon as her mother started to pull the car away from the curb. Six weeks of loss tumbled out in an avalanche of weeping.

Mrs. Hinds pulled into a parking space and turned off the engine. Pulling her daughter into her arms she stroked her hair and tried to speak words of comfort to her. "Honey, let it out."

Elaine's sobs grew louder and her body involuntarily shook. "Why? Mom, how much more?"

Mrs. Hinds hugged Elaine tighter before she responded. "I don't know, Hon, I just don't know." Elaine and her mother sat in the front seat of the station wagon for what seemed like an eternity.

With her mother's arms wrapped around her, Elaine tried to make sense of her life's circumstances. She began to regain her composure and moved back to the passenger's side of the car. "Mom, I have to pull myself back together. I don't want Albert to see me fall apart. Let's take the long way home."

The older woman wiped away her own tears before responding. "We'll ride through the park and then down by the river." She reached into her purse for the small wallet size packet of tissues. "Here, Honey."

Elaine gratefully accepted the tissues, wiped her eyes, and took a deep breath. "Do you think we're strong enough?" She found herself no longer asking if she and Al would get through one event because the tragedies kept coming.

Her mother did not hesitate to answer. "Yes. The love you have for each other will not change. You'll find the strength you need and solutions to your problems because of that love. You're physically worn down. Give yourself time to recuperate."

Elaine looked doubtfully out the windshield. "That's a nice, neat answer, Mom."

"It's the only one that is real. God never promised you an easy life, he just promised life." The older woman looked sadly at her daughter and then began the orchestrated extra, long drive home.

Elaine refocused her attention beyond the glass in front of her. "I hope Al didn't have a difficult first night." She turned her head to look out the passenger window and the hospital fell from view. The conversation between the women became perfunctory until the car pulled into the driveway an hour later.

"Elaine, dad and I will stay all day. You will have plenty of help. Please, rest." Mrs. Hinds gripped the steering wheel tightly.

"Thanks, Mom. I wonder how Al's first night home went?" Elaine began to replace her feelings of loss with a focus on her husband's recovery.

Elaine was not aware yet, of the intensity of the headaches

Al was experiencing. Mr. Hinds had mentioned it to his wife in an early morning phone call she made from the hospital, but they both agreed to wait until Elaine was home to decide how much she could handle. For his part, Al wanted to be alert when she came home so that he could comfort her, but as he placed the protective goggles over the bandaged eyes that morning, he wondered if he would be able to last an extended amount of time without more codeine.

By memory, he found his way to the master bath and flipped the switch he knew was on the left out of habit. He heard the soft click of the switch and snorted sarcastically.

What am I doing?

After using the bathroom, he walked back into the bedroom counting his steps to his dresser to find a shirt and boxers. His headache drummed steadily.

I've got to find new ways to overcome this constant pain without medication. It can't last forever.

He counted down three drawers, opened one and felt for the T-shirts and boxers. Pulling each one out, he left both hanging off the edge of the drawer.

I hope I don't look ridiculous. I have no idea what color this shirt is. Maybe I'll get lucky and it will be a white one.

He found the bottom edge of the fresh shirt, opened it and then carefully and slowly pulled the clothing over his head easing both arms in. Leaning on the dresser for support, he realized even without a pounding headache, bending to dress in a standing position was still a challenge.

I have to get a system down for my clothes. I don't want Elaine dressing me. I'll throw on my bathrobe and deal with the jeans later.

Al felt around for the sturdy cane the hospital sent him home with. He knew he had brought it into the bedroom yesterday, but could not remember where he had put it. Arms waving in front of him, Al walked to the closet in the master bedroom, felt for the hook inside on the left and found his robe still hung where he had left it two months ago. Gingerly, he slipped each arm into the thin cotton, grateful he hadn't replaced this old robe with a new one and stubbed his toe on the cane knocking it over and hurting his new skin.

The smell of freshly brewing coffee wafted into the bedroom as he stepped into the old slippers that were always near his robe. Al decided to leave the cane on the floor inside the closet and take his chances on the obstacle course waiting for him in the living room. Walking out of the bedroom into the hallway he knew immediately he should have taken it with him.

Mr. Hinds looked up from his plate and saw the hunched over figure navigating into the kitchen. "We have coffee cake, cereal or I can make eggs. What would you like?"

Albert in his high chair saw his dad approaching and tried to call out around cheeks full of banana. "Da."

Al heard the garbled voice of his son as he kicked toys in front of him. "Good morning to you too, Albert." He was getting close to the breakfast bar, reached in front, found the back of a chair, and gingerly edged his way around to sit. "Some tea would be good, Dad." Al realized he had no idea what time it was. "Can we keep the radio on low in the kitchen? I keep track of my day that way."

Mr. Hinds pulled the portable radio down from the top of the fridge where Ronnie placed it yesterday and put it on the counter in front of Al. "Here you go. Music would be good."

Al had been used to listening to news stations, but as he ran his hand over the twelve by eight black box, he found a rock station. A tune from the top forty came on in a sedated volume, bringing back the feeling of the previous summer. Immediately images of himself, Elaine and the baby on the sand in Point Pleasant Beach gave him a minuscule amount of relief from his headache. Little Albert had no fear of the water on their day trip, screaming delightfully as his father dipped him up and down into the surf. Elaine sat comfortably back on her elbows, smiling and digging her toes into the warm sand and watching her two men.

Mr. Hinds poured Al a cup of tea and placed it in front of Al and noticed how quiet he had become. "Where did you go? Are

(102)

you caught up in the music? Tea is right in front of you."

Al pushed the radio toward his father-in-law. "Dad, can you put this next to the stove? I need some distance from the speaker." He felt for the cup in front of him, grateful that it was not too hot. "I'll need the Timoptic drops this morning. The drops helped to relieve some of the pressure last night."

Al took a sip of his tea and carefully placed the cup on the counter, listening as he heard his father-in-law walk to the refrigerator for the bag of medication kept out of Albert's reach. The older man's gait had grown familiar to Al. He had never noticed how Mr. Hinds favored his left side, relying on his right to carry the extra weight he had put on in recent years.

Al lifted his goggles off and placed them to the left of his teacup inadvertently tapping the mug. The metallic sound the goggles made created a scene in his mind of himself looking like a bandaged Clark Kent. "Dad, is this too gruesome for you or the little guy?" He stopped before proceeding any further.

Mr. Hinds placed the bottle in Al's free left hand. "Are you serious? Son, you were a mess right after the accident, now you look normal. Relax. Do what you have to do. I got Albert under control with the new toys the man from the Stanley Company dropped off with Elaine's order." He glanced over at the toddler in his high chair, eating banana pieces and banging together the three toddler-sized pieces of a plastic orange giraffe toy.

Al began to lift off the bandages covering his right eye with one hand, still holding the bottle of drops in the other. Mr. Hinds saw Al's white eye exposed and compassion flooded through him. No longer visible was the deep warm brown color his daughter had found so compelling. There was no pupil or iris, just a white film devoid of color.

Mr. Hinds turned back to the baby and saw the kitchen door open behind the high chair. Elaine walked slowly inside followed by Mrs. Hinds.

"Hi, Sweetheart." Mr. Hinds kissed her on the cheek.

"Hi, Dad." Elaine looked past her father and saw Al replacing the bandages on his right eye. "Hi, Al?" She watched as

(103)

he took care of his own needs. "How are you doing?"

Humbled that Elaine was still thinking about him after all she had been through, he couldn't immediately answer her and instead placed his goggles back over his eyes. "How are *you?*"

Silently she walked over to the highchair and touched her son's hair. Albert was transfixed by his giraffe until he felt her touch. "Mama."

Elaine smiled down at Albert. "How do you like having your dad home? The baby looked over at Al and then went back to playing and sporadically eating.

Elaine walked around the end of the breakfast bar and reached for Al's hand. The second he felt her move near him and then touch his hand he sprung temporarily from the vise grip of pain the headaches and healing burn tissue still held him in.

Al fought past the lump in his throat to speak. "I was so worried about you. I am so sorry."

Elaine cut him off. "Al, it wasn't meant to be." She closed her eyes and then opened them slowly. "I'm tired and need to lie down for a while, but first I want to hear how your night was."

Al shook himself free from the shock of his wife's strength. "I slept through the night with the help of codeine but the drumming in my head has been building. The drops are helping." He squeezed her hand and wondered if he should continue. "It's glaucoma. We knew this would happen but I didn't think it would be on the first day home." Al paused briefly before changing the subject. "I'm worried about you."

Glad to focus on Al's recovery instead of her own, Elaine took control. "After I rest I'll call Dr. Westmont and see what he thinks about the glaucoma." She held his hand a little tighter.

Mrs. Hinds looked over at her weary daughter. "It might be a good idea if both of you rest after Al has something to eat."

Al was grateful to have the chance to be alone with his wife, but had to admit that he also wanted to return to the bed he had just climbed out of. "She's right, Elaine. You go ahead. I'll be finished in a couple of minutes." The smell of toast was inviting to him in spite of the pounding in his head.

Mr. Hinds stood on the other side of the breakfast bar. "Eat as much as you can, Son. You need to keep up your strength and your medication should not be taken on an empty stomach. I have to get to work. I'll call you later and see how everyone is."

Elaine spoke and felt a lump form in her throat. "Thanks, Dad. Can you bring me up to speed on Al's medication disbursement before you leave?

"Elaine, I can let you know." Al felt his frustration grow. He needed to regain control over his existence and unconsciously expressed this when he removed his hand from hers. "Please, go lie down. Your mom can take care of the baby and I'm fine. I'll tell her the medications I took already, and she can start the log we're supposed to keep."

Elaine relented and wearily pushed herself up off the breakfast bar stool. An hour later she watched him slowly approach the bed she had taken refuge in.

She sat up on her elbow. "How do you feel about using the cane?" She watched how gingerly as he moved to the bed without it.

"To be honest, the cane is more for physical support right now. I feel a little weak from the headache." He slowly came closer to the bed as Elaine saw the sturdy metal cane usually given to patients with physical limitations hung where she had left it after finding it on their closet floor. "I don't think the folding cane for people without sight would help me right now." He found the edge of the bed and eased himself on the pillows Elaine had left in place for him. "Sorry the bed wasn't made for you."

She smiled at the familiarity that was returning to them. "I've missed you, Al."

Al reached for her hand and held it tightly. "Me too." He breathed out deeply and tried to relax.

Elaine knew the headache was worse than he was admitting. "When was your last pill?"

Al tried to articulate around the pain. "Last night." Each thrum of his headache tested his resilience of limiting his pain medication. "I want to see Dr. Westmont tomorrow. I'm worried that the headaches are starting so soon. It wasn't supposed to be this fast." His expression of doubt on his release from the hospital felt more like a confession he needed to purge to Elaine. "Maybe I should have stayed another week in the hospital or maybe it's the stress of coming home that I can't handle yet." Al breathed deeply. "I don't know if that is the cause or if this would have happened in the hospital." The phone rang on the nightstand next to Al and he moaned in reaction. "Oh, God. Why is that thing so loud?" He lay in his misery and reached for the phone, dragging the handset and cord across him to Elaine.

She reached up to grasp the mustard colored handset, catching it as Al let it fall loosely from his grip. A woman's voice called out for someone to answer her. "Hello? Is anyone there?"

Elaine recognized Rose Plevier. "Hi, Mom."

Rose Plevier had been told about Elaine's miscarriage by Helen Hinds last night. "Hello, Dear. How are you?"

Elaine glanced over at her sick husband. "Tired. Mom, Al is having a headache that is only growing worse. We're going to call Dr. Westmont. We were wondering if you or Fenna could watch Albert while we are at the appointment?"

On the other end of the phone, Rose brought her hand to her mouth before continuing. "Elaine, maybe it would be better if we took him so that you can rest. You need to regain your strength." Rose squeezed her eyes shut tightly, willing the tears and the growing lump in her throat to subside.

Elaine's heart warmed knowing Rose was going through her own torment watching her son work at recovering. "Mom, thank you, but I'll call you back as soon as I talk to Dr. Westmont. It will help us both to know that Albert is happy with his grandma or his aunt."

"We'll do whatever you need." Rose stood frozen. "Please take care of yourself too."

"I will, Mom, I promise." Elaine said good-bye and reached across Al to replace the handset back in its cradle. "I have to get Dr. Westmont's number from the file. I'll call him from the kitchen while I get you some codeine and the Diamox drops." She didn't give Al the opportunity for a discussion or a response.

Watching his agonizingly slow movements left her more determined to convince the doctor of the need for possible re-admittance to the hospital. She sat on the edge of the bed and watched his body, stiff with reaction to the pain of the headaches and burns. Elaine allowed her mind to drift to what once was, what could have been, and finally to what would be now.

Al hadn't tried to say anything else. The guilt that his wife had to take care of him, coupled with the fact that he was almost paralyzed by the migraine, deposited him into a black void of nothingness, compliments of the codeine.

Elaine left the bedroom and walked into the living room, her mother looked up in surprise. "Shouldn't you be lying down?"

"Mom, Al's headache is growing. The doctors warned us about secondary glaucoma. I have to call Dr. Westmont." Elaine found her purse on the kitchen counter and searched inside for the office number as she spoke to her mother. "The doctor wanted to wait to do the surgery, trying to give his body more time to heal, but I don't know. Unless his medication is increased, he may have to go back into the hospital."

Elaine called the office and to her surprise was able to speak to Dr. Westmont immediately. She spent the next ten minutes on the phone trying to convince the doctor to readmit her husband for reevaluation on the immediate necessity for surgery.

She hung up the phone and turned to her mother. "He agreed to see him in the morning at the hospital and to do an evaluation as an outpatient. I have to get Al his medication." She turned to her silent mother as she sorted through the pill bottles on top of the fridge. "Mom thank you for your help and everything else. I couldn't do this without you. I'm just not up to chasing the little guy."

Mrs. Hinds smiled weakly at her weary daughter. "Dad and I will do whatever we can." She looked at her grandson pushing cars on the gold carpet. "He seems pretty content with me right now. I'll bundle him up and take him for a stroller ride after lunch."

(107)

Elaine walked back to the bedroom. "Al, I have the codeine and Diamox drops. I'll get some water and be right back."

Once in the bathroom, Elaine saw the maternity vitamins still on the sink next to her toothbrush. Trying to ignore them, she quickly filled a small plastic bathroom cup with water and walked into the bedroom.

"I'm putting the pill in your left hand." She let the cup touch his right fingers and he gingerly wrapped his hand around it.

Shaking herself, she got up, walked to her side of the bed and laid down next to her husband. They spent the rest of the day and evening in the master bedroom, mustering the strength to recover from the last several days and to face the doctor's appointment.

The next day Elaine relented and allowed her father to take Al to his appointment. Relieved that she had decided to stay home eased Al's guilt and he began to lose himself in the escalating pain behind his right eye. The car ride was an exercise in agony.

During the appointment at the hospital, Dr. Westmont confirmed secondary glaucoma caused by the fluid that normally drains from the eye building up around the optic nerve. The scarring damage done to the tear ducts by the sodium hydroxide had closed the ducts in the right eye completely now. The eye had become swollen and the retina and optic nerve had begun to tear in not only the right eye but also the left.

"The pressure in the right eye is going to become steadily worse over the next several weeks. I'm reluctant to perform the surgery due to the proximity of the date of the initial injury. We will increase the dosage and frequency of medications to get you through until we can perform another surgery." Dr. Westmont interpreted Al's stony expression as the admission of more pain. He put down the eye model he had been using to explain the scenario more clearly to Mr. Hinds and waited for a reaction from either of them. "We want to hold out as long as possible for the surgery."

Mr. Hinds stopped waiting for Al to speak. "He needs a date to focus on so he can work through the pain." He looked over at Al whose expression suddenly broke.

"What is this crap?" Al's angry outburst fed the thrumming in his head. "This is worse than during the hospital stay. Get me under the knife now!"

"You were on more medication in the hospital, and the condition is now progressing quickly. Let's try to wait at least a week." Dr. Westmont's voice took on a pleading tone as he sympathized and tried to remain professional.

Al was still in the elevated exam chair before he spoke. "I never thanked you for saving my eyes, but I need this pain to end."

Dr. Westmont began to lower the exam chair and then aided his patient to his feet. "You're right where you should be in your recovery."

The car ride home from the office was silent. Al began to feel the effects from the dose of narcotics Dr. Westmont's nurse had given him almost the second the car began to move. When two men arrived home, Elaine was briefed on Al's condition, and the pain he would have to endure while waiting for clearance on the procedure to alleviate it. She watched him suffer, alone in the void of pain that had become his existence, for another week. For herself, she sought the comfort required to deal with the miscarriage from her mother. One day Mrs. Hinds arrived after work to help and found Elaine crying at the kitchen counter.

Mrs. Hinds wrapped her arms around her. "Hon, I'm here. Where's Albert?"

Elaine wiped her face with a tissue before answering in short responses. "He and Al are both sleeping. Al took codeine an hour ago and is getting some relief from the pain. It has moved passed the intensity of a migraine. He is really suffering." She brought her hands to her face, wiping away more tears.

Mrs. Hinds sat down and hoped she could find the right words of comfort. "You'll get through this, I promise."

Elaine let herself release the emotions. "Mom, I'm so tired. I'm just so tired. What about the family Al and I wanted? What about our plans for our life together? We both wanted this baby so much." She cried steadily while her mother held her.

Mrs. Hinds let Elaine cry until she was ready to stop. "You still have your family, and you and Al do not have to let go of your dreams for the future. Some of what you're feeling could also be your body readjusting. Honey, your hormones, and emotions have been on a roller coaster ride the last two months. Cry all you want with me."

She leaned into her mother gratefully. "It's hard to believe our lives will ever be normal."

She had been trying not to think past five-minute intervals even though Thanksgiving loomed three days away. The holiday Al had worked so hard to be home for would pass by unnoticed by him. What was supposed to be a time of gratitude for life would be clouded with the constant overwhelming pain he found himself trapped in.

The week after Thanksgiving, Elaine heard a pounding noise coming from the master bath. She walked through the bedroom and knocked on the closed door. "Al?" She opened the door to find her husband pounding his head against the linoleum floor from the intense pain that had continued growing over the last week. "Al! What are you doing?"

Al barely heard her. "I can take being blind, but I can't take the pain." Al rolled onto his left side curling into the fetal position.

The temporary solution of Valium, codeine or mild doses of morphine was not working. The Diamox and Timoptic diuretics that controlled the swelling only until the permanent surgical solutions had reached their effective end.

Panic came over Elaine. "Al, for God's sake, you're going to kill yourself doing that!" Leaving her husband on the bathroom floor, she ran to the bedside phone and called Dr. Westmont.

She practically screamed into the phone. "Something has to be done today. We're going to the hospital." Elaine finished the phone call after confirming the doctor would meet them in the emergency room.

Elaine ran back to the master bath. "Al, we're going to the hospital. Ronnie's still here. She can stay with Albert until Mom and Dad both get off work."

Al pulled himself up off the floor with a Herculean effort and clung to the door frame as Elaine ran into the living room to speak to Ronnie and say goodbye to their toddler. Al collapsed across the backseat of the car wanting only for the ride to end and the oblivion of more drugs to take effect.

Five minutes from the hospital Al finally spoke. "Elaine, can you tell me how far away we are? How much longer? How many minutes?" Déjà vu came over him in the form of inescapable, excruciating pain, and waiting for relief.

"We're pulling up to the entrance now." Elaine stopped the car, got out and opened Al's door. He practically crawled out, hunched over and reached for her arm to walk through the double doors that swung inward, welcoming them back to prison after being on the run.

Al was operated on immediately. Dr. Westmont made a slit in each eye to drain the fluid and relieve the pressure. Elaine sat, once again, in the unforgiving orange plastic chairs and waited. Sooner than she expected, a voice she recognized called her.

"Mrs. Plevier?" Dr. Westmont stood in front of the nurse's station looking tired and old.

Elaine rose quickly and walked over to him. "How is he?"

"He came through the procedure fine. He's going to be medicated for the rest of the night. I would prefer that he did not have any visitors until tomorrow." Dr. Westmont yawned widely slightly moved the wire frame glasses and blinked before speaking. "He will wake up tomorrow without a headache."

Elaine felt her face relax. "Thank you. I'll call the nurses station to check on him." Her ritual had begun.

Doctor Westmont nodded and smiled slightly before leaving. Elaine wished she had brought someone along to drive with, but no one was available at that time of the day. Everyone was working and living their lives. Turning around slowly, she returned to the plastic chair to gather her thoughts before she started the hour drive home.

(111)

I have to get used to this. I'm a seasoned veteran of hospitals now.

After this last thought, she picked up her purse, walked down the hallway, out the double doors and into the parking lot. She turned to look back toward the upper floors of the hospital and repeated the same silent prayer from two months ago.

Come back to us, Al. Just live.

Chapter IX: The Business of Life

*D*uring the early morning hours, the next day, before the sedatives completely dissipated, Al dreamed of babies. Ten of them were crowded together and sitting on a rug in a white room looking up at him with imploring eyes. In the middle was Albert who, at the sight of his father, broke into a smile and held his hands up high. He could see every detail of Albert's face and body with his chubby little hands that were just learning how to play. Al reached down and picked Albert up off the carpet he became a newborn held closely in his father's arms for the first time. The scene became the day of his birth and Al looked up from the chair where he sat holding his first son for the first time and watched Elaine rest in the bed after twenty hours of labor.

Elation grew inside Al as thoughts of Little League and Yankee games formed in his imagination. The new baby boy was so tiny and the possibilities for his life were endless. Al turned his head toward the door and saw his mother-in-law and father-in-law rush breathlessly into the room from a weekend retreat in Mystic Connecticut. He smiled broadly at them tried to adjust the baby so his grandparents could get a better view but felt resistance. Al struggled gently but was confused on how the little bundle could fight him.

He began to panic as he awoke rapidly from the dream, confused as to where he was and why the darkness. "Hello?" Al heard his scratchy voice, smelled antiseptic, heard machines beeping and knew he was in a hospital. Fear washed over him. "Mary? Is that you?"

"Sorry to disappoint you, Al, it's me." Elaine sat near him.

Al breathed a sigh of relief. "Let's get out of here." He gave no thought to the heaviness in his arms caused by the drugs that had kept him sedated for the last twenty hours or the emergency surgery he had endured. He had even forgotten the pain of yesterday.

"Relax. Don't you remember why you're here?" Elaine looked at him incredulously and couldn't believe the first words he spoke were not of relief.

"No. I don't know." Orientation began to leave him and confusion set in. "When did I get here?"

"Al, it's December 4. You came in yesterday and had surgery to relieve the glaucoma." Elaine touched his left hand and squeezed gently. "Do you want a sip of water?"

Al now realized that his head was not pounding. The relief suddenly exhausted him. "No. Are we alone?"

"No. You have two roommates, but you will only be here for a day or two. Dr. Westmont wants you to recover at home." Elaine looked at her husband's relaxed face.

"I'm so tired. I could sleep for a week. Wait. Did you say December 4?" Al could feel a faint pressure in his right eye. It was almost as if to remind him the condition still existed. "I'm sorry. I guess you didn't have much of a birthday."

She was touched that he was able to think of her December 2 birthday after what he went through. "Get well. That's your gift to me this year."

He relaxed heavily into the pillow. "My head is good now, but I still feel the pain in the eyeball."

Elaine looked over his face carefully. "You have to tell the doctor. From now on he has to know how bad or how good you feel if there is going to be a real chance to salvage your sight in the future."

"Agreed." A very small smile at the corners of Al's mouth began to appear. "I can think." He gingerly turned his head from side to side testing to see if the unbearable pain would return. "What happened to the last couple of weeks? I don't remember much beyond living from one pain pill to the next."

Elaine held his hand. "It was bad for you. We were all in survivor mode."

Melancholy washed over him and the small smile faded slowly. "I wanted to get home for Thanksgiving so badly and I missed it anyway. I don't even remember the day. I'm sorry. I should not have put you through the last couple of weeks. I should have stayed at Overlook."

Elaine squeezed his hand to comfort both of them. "We didn't have a dinner. Mom brought over some food on plates and we had dessert later that day." She paused. "I know we were working toward a small celebration with family but I think our expectations were unrealistic. We have to work within the parameters we are dealing with. The important thing is you will be home in a day or two."

Elaine was right. Three days later the two made the drive home, without the drama of the first trip. He was kept on Diamox and Timoptic to keep the pressure in his eyes from building and had a prescription available for Valium and Codeine if any pain developed. The surgery helped considerably, but both Al and Elaine knew the pressure and the pain would build once more. He mentally prepared himself for more eye surgery and continued to adapt to a world without sight.

During the drive, home Al wanted desperately to broach the subject of the lost baby. "Elaine, I'm so sorry I couldn't drive you to the hospital." The guilt he felt was overwhelming.

Elaine was still dealing with her feelings about the miscarriage, but did not want to discuss it. "We talked about this.

The baby wasn't meant to be."

Al refused to let the enormity of the loss go unspoken. "Sweetheart, we didn't talk about this." Al took a breath before continuing. "You have had a tremendous amount of stress coupled with all the burdens of the daily management of our life. The combination of those two things is too much for most people, let alone a pregnant woman."

Elaine knew that since Al was feeling better, talking about the miscarriage could no longer be avoided. "That baby meant the world to me. I won't lie to you, Al."

He relaxed a little feeling that as long as the truth was before them. "Me too. I can't imagine what you went through alone. I should have been there for you."

The emotions that led to Elaine breaking down after the miscarriage had been healing. "You're here for me now."

The car pulled onto the familiar gravel and Al relaxed even further. "Elaine, I love you." The two were silent as the car came to a stop. "I feel really good, except for the burns. I can even deal with that now that my head doesn't feel like knives are being jabbed into my skull. Let me start to find my way around the yard. I'll get the mail and enjoy the fresh air." He felt the cold air hit his healing scar tissue the second he stepped out of the car and realized he might have made a mistake. "You might want to keep an eye on me."

"Are you sure you're up to this?" She watched him move away from the car.

"I feel good." Al started toward the mailbox with a slow shuffling gait.

"You need your cane, hold on a minute." She opened the back door of the car, retrieved the cane and walked toward her husband.

Al heard Elaine approaching on the gravel and held out his hand. "Thanks. You're always right." Without hesitation, he grabbed the cane, turned around and started to where he believed the mailbox would be. He poked the cane in front of him to make sure he was still on the gravel driveway.

On this second homecoming from Overlook Hospital Al felt, physically, a bit more in control. He calculated that everything, including navigating his own home and yard, would take him four times longer to learn and complete. His engineering background gave him the perspective to assume that once he learned and completed a task, it would take less time on further attempts. Through experience during his first stay at Overlook, he realized that the world within his control was now his two-foot reach to the front, back, right and left of where he stood. This sphere creates an eight-foot world that travels with him as he interacts with the world of the sighted. He stepped out of the car that morning determined in any small way to prove to his wife and to himself that he would not be a burden. He felt himself rising above the healing, burn tissue of his body that was itching, painful, raw and ever-present.

Elaine looked at her husband's awkward movements and yelled at him. "We have to get the Blind Commission to teach you how to use that thing. You're going to trip."

Al felt defiance rise to the surface. "Not a chance." The surface grew harder as he poked along with his cane.

"You're not even halfway. Don't forget to account for the bend in the driveway." She wondered how much longer this test of her patience would take as she glanced at her watch and thought of all the chores inside the house that awaited her.

"I got it. I can tell the difference between the grass, the dirt and the road." He moved forward, determined to bring some sense of productivity to his recovery. Each step had an effect on both his healing tissue and the pressure still behind his eye, but he ignored both. He had left the hospital that morning without the aid of a narcotic for the drive home feeling like he was gaining some control over his recovery process.

I've got to have more patience with him as he gains his independence back. "Don't forget to account for the change in your stride." She glances at her watch.

Al secretly hoped Elaine would find something to do inside. "Thanks for keeping an eye on me this first time. Where's

(117)

Jayne Kelly

the mailbox?"

"Dead ahead about ten feet on the left." Elaine continued to watch the efforts of the man she loved with admiration. *I have to call the Blind Commission this afternoon. I won't have the time to teach him navigating around the property and take care of the baby. He can do this alone with the proper training. He already adjusted to the car or maybe he knows better than to complain. He never said a word the entire trip home.* Elaine decided to trust him and turned away in time to hear a smack of metal against something.

"Got it!" Al could tell he had hit wood and believed it to be the post the mailbox sat on.

She smiled and worked a sarcastic answer to keep his spirits up. "Nice try, but that's the fence post you were supposed to take out last spring. The mailbox is two more feet." Elaine watched Al travel the last two feet of his journey and hit the mailbox hard with the cane."

"Thanks." He hoped his success would send her inside.

It worked. "I'm going in. Yell if you get stuck."

Al waved in the direction of her voice as he heard the back door close. *Damn it's cold out here. I got the mail, so I'll turn around and go back where I came from. Was it 50 or 40 steps? That can't be right. I stopped and started a couple times.* Al stood still to regain his bearings and think. *The bend will go the other way now and I'll go slow until I whack the car. I'll know exactly where I am then because she has been parking in the same place now that I'm home and the MG isn't in the way.* He continued to move down the driveway toward what he thought was the direction of the back door still clutching the mail in his healing right hand.

Five minutes later Elaine stuck her head out the door. "How about if I come down the driveway and get you?"

Al yelled back to his wife. "Like a two-year-old? No thanks. Just tell me how close I am." Al continued to shuffle and poke with the cane until he hit something in front of him.

Elaine held the door open and watched his progress. "Nice try but, that's the car. Come in before you freeze."

(118)

"Everything is going to take me longer even after I map out the house and yard in my head." Al followed her voice and held the back door open for her. After he was in the kitchen, he decided to try his luck at finding a drinking glass. He first found the sink, then the cabinet that held the glasses and then turned around and negotiated his way to the refrigerator. Elaine stood at the counter as she flipped through the mail and watched.

"Do you want me to get something for you?" She dropped the mail on the counter.

Al stopped in the middle of walking. "I'm fine." He regretted his snotty tone the minute it was out of his mouth. "You have enough to do. Why don't you relax while Ronnie is still here?" He began to fish around inside the fridge to become acquainted with the location of its contents.

Elaine rolled her eyes. "If you're trying to get rid of me, just say so."

Al waited until he heard her walk across the living room, grabbed the container on the left of the top shelf and walked over to the counter to pour a glass with the orange juice he thought he chose. He lifted the glass and took a large sip and almost spit milk across the kitchen.

"Bleck!" He followed the counter around, running his right hand lightly across its edge and poured the rest of the glass of milk into the sink. As he rinsed the glass, Ronnie came in.

"What's wrong?" Ronnie walked in with her coat already on, preparing to escape before Elaine changed her mind.

"I grabbed the milk instead of the OJ." He filled his glass with water and rinsed his mouth without the required gentleness. His healing lips cracked and he recoiled slightly.

She let out an annoyed breath. "I thought you hurt yourself by the sound you made. You guys should mark the containers." Ronnie looked at Al and pictured his nose on a container of juice. "Maybe I better bring my own food over for a while. I don't want to drink something where your nose has been." Smiling and laughing, Ronnie turned and walked toward the door.

Al snickered behind her. "It might be worth grossing you

out to get you to stop sponging food out of my fridge."

Ronnie stopped short at the back door laughing. "I think I might live longer if I bring my own. Elaine's cooking is marginal and you can't cook with or without sight."

"You got that right on all points." Al put down his glass as he heard Elaine enter the kitchen.

"What are you doing?" Elaine went to the fridge.

Al rinsed his mouth one more time before responding. "Trying to get the taste of milk out of my mouth. I thought I grabbed the orange juice."

"You shouldn't be drinking orange juice. The acid will bother your mouth and hurt your lips." She looked over the contents.

Al opened his mouth and then spoke. "We need to mark the containers in the fridge like we do for my medication, Sweetie. Do we have any paper clips?" Al put the glass down and started to fumble through the first drawer he found.

"Here." Elaine reached in a drawer next to the fridge and pulled out a few paper clips. "I'll put a paper clip or a piece of tape on the orange juice and leave the milk alone." Elaine reached into the fridge, put a paper clip on the container and shut the door firmly.

As she turned to leave Al grabbed her around the waist. Surprised, Elaine stood still as her husband, still unable to kiss his wife, hugged her as tightly as his limitations permitted. "I miss you too, Al. You're healing every day."

He released her and tried to get a drink. "It's good to be home. The smell of our home and the river are so comforting. I was in so much pain I didn't notice."

Moving over to the breakfast bar, Elaine changed the mood in the kitchen by pulling an envelope from the mail she had dropped in a pile on the counter. She noticed it was from the state and knew immediately that it had to be the check she had been waiting for.

Relieved, she looked over at her husband and wondered if he had enough energy left to talk about money. "Al, I need to talk you about financial decisions we need to make. I thought since you're feeling better, it would be a good time."

"Let's get it over with." He stood next to the sink shifting his weight from one foot to the other and then walked toward Elaine's voice running his right hand along the counter for orientation.

Elaine watched his movements with trepidation but continued the discussion. "Do you remember when my father brought up the idea of contacting an attorney?" Elaine opened the envelope as she spoke.

Al walked into a chair and sat down. "That was the last I heard about it. So, what have *we* decided?"

Elaine's tone changed to one of irritation. "This conversation isn't to bring you up to speed on what I've decided, you need to catch up on what has transpired while you were in pain and trying to survive." Elaine watched the annoyed look on Al's face and plunged forward. "I did hear from the attorney, Art Bayplaza. He came to the house and spent an hour or so explaining our position and setting the lawsuit in motion."

Al's look of annoyance turned to surprise. "A house visit by a lawyer? We must have a great case." He has been so caught up in his health issues, he had forgotten Elaine was managing one of the marital takes she hated and had previously left to him. "How are we making out with paying the bills? I'm sorry to ask you to do it."

"I'm getting used to it." Elaine gave this as an explanation for doing a chore she abhorred. "Don't get your hopes up with the case. I think the lawyer came out to the house because I couldn't get to him while I was spending time at the hospital." Elaine took a sip of her coffee. "The visit was about five weeks after you were hurt, and he knew I did not have the time or the emotional fortitude to make an office appointment." She burrowed through the papers in the folder looking for something specific. "He is also a very good friend of Bob Sylvania and you know how tight Bob and dad are." Elaine thought about the lifelong friendship between the two.

Al drummed his fingers. "What do we do next?"

(121)

Elaine walked around the breakfast bar and retrieved a manila folder from a drawer. "I filed for the Worker's Compensation checks with Mr. Bayplaza's help. I thought that was automatic. I didn't realize I had to file for more than the hospital repayment and the payment for the nurses provided by them."

Al stopped drumming his fingers and felt anger rise in him at the thought of Worker's Compensation and A&K. "Wait. We have the private policy that covers us and gives income if I get hurt. Does the lawyer know that?"

Elaine continued. "Yes. It was a choice for us. We chose Worker's Compensation. We can't have both policies kick in at once so we thought it would be better to go with the state."

Al spoke flippantly. "I assumed the company would take care of that kind of paperwork stuff. Guess I assumed too much about everything. Did A&K file the medical paperwork for us?"

Elaine looked at her husband's body language and knew he was revisiting the anger he held for both the plant and himself. "Yes, upper management had to do the paperwork for the medical the night you were brought in. The hospital asked for the insurance cards immediately. The hospital and any subsequent medical expenses will be 100% covered including mileage and gas to and from the hospital and doctor's visits."

"Did you file the Worker's Comp claim?" Al thought about the claims that had come across his desk at the plant and how he never hesitated to fill out the forms and forward them to the necessary agency or the plant's front office.

He sat across from his wife and wondered where the mercy was with the people in charge of the employees he was no longer capable of taking care of. Who would look out for them or the residual effects upon his own family?

Elaine went through the timeline of events. "I filed two weeks after your accident. I couldn't think clearly before then. The good news is that it Worker's Compensation payments are retroactive from the day you were hurt, but the bad news is that you were awarded only $112.00 per week." Elaine had opened the envelope.

Al dropped his head down and talked to his lap. "We have to do some financial scrambling. We would do better with my private plan."

Elaine shook her head. "No, this is a little better."

Al lifted his head and folded his hands in front of him. "I take it we are not moving to Rainbow Lake?" Al let himself reminisce about the move to a bigger and more modern home for which he and Elaine had a contract on and a closing date solidified shortly before he was hurt.

"We were turned down for the mortgage after the bank found out about the decrease in income." Elaine placed the check on the counter while she opened the folder.

Al shook his head slowly with sadness. "I knew things must have been on hold. I'm sorry I couldn't help out with the decisions. I can do some of that for you now." Overwhelmed with guilt his triumphant trip to the mailbox suddenly seemed trivial.

Elaine watched Al's reaction. "There's pretzels on the counter." Elaine and Al grabbed a few of the pretzels before she continued. "Our finances are always going to have to be negotiated through." Silence enveloped them and then Elaine spoke. "We've planned our life together since high school. I don't see any reason for us to let our new circumstances change that."

"Absolutely. We're going to continue with our life plans." Al felt the determination he used to survive the hospital rise inside him. "Let's get all this laid out so we can at least figure out where we are financially. I'll need time to mull this over."

Elaine moved forward. "Since the bank notified us of the cancelation of the mortgage on the new house, the next call I made was to the agent representing the seller to expedite the return of our deposit." Elaine felt her own anger swell inside her and stopped to take a sip of the coffee her sister had made to regain her composure. "The sellers don't want to give us back our deposit willingly so I had to contact our real estate lawyer to file a claim against the sellers. To quote the seller: "Sorry for your troubles but we have problems of our own." Elaine stopped short.

"What!" He sat perfectly still and rigid as Elaine dropped

(123)

the financial bomb on him.

She continued in a monotone as their dark financial future revisited itself on her. "The buyers of this house were kind enough to back out of the contract after the realtor explained the circumstances. The contract for this house hadn't made it through attorney review." Elaine let all the information she had given Al sink in before she continued. "There are good people in the world."

He was still considering the potential loss of the deposit money on the Rainbow Lake house. "Isn't that guy who owns the Rainbow Lake house a doctor?" He felt a cold weight in the pit of his stomach.

Elaine almost spit the word out. "Yes." She twisted a strand of blond hair around her left index finger. "I thought he would have compassion or, at the very least, an understanding that this situation was out of our control, but I turned it over to the lawyer. We can't reason with them so let the lawyer fight it out."

Al began to alternately fold his hands over one another as he tried to make sense out of the latest financial setback. "What did the lawyer say our chances are?"

"The usual threats are going back and forth, but he believes that legally the seller cannot hold onto the deposit. We can put a lean on the property and that will hold up any pending sale from a new buyer." She watched a look of relief spread across Al's face and reached across the counter and put her hands over his.

He slipped out from her touch, rose from the stool and shifted his weight from one foot to the other. "Man, people kick you when you're down."

Elaine found another opening she was looking for. "I guess we can either lie down and take it or get up and continue to fight. Do you feel you're up for a larger fight?"

"You mean the lawsuit?" He continued to shift from one foot to the other.

Elaine heard the mix of anger, frustration, and helplessness in his voice and hoped the discussion would leave him feeling empowered. "You need to know where we stand. The Worker's

Comp case and the lawsuit are two different matters. The paperwork is a career in and of itself." The exasperation Elaine had been overwhelmed with was finally being shared with her husband, and she could not contain the relief in her voice. "We can't sue A&K because, under New Jersey law, the company is covered with Worker's Compensation." She repeated her earlier summary. "The Worker's Comp covered the hospitalization 100%, and any subsequent care involved. It also reimbursed a percentage of the mileage for driving back and forth to the hospital and to doctors' visits. Worker's Comp estimates that the bills, over the next twenty years, could run into the hundreds of thousands of dollars." She paused as Al made a low whistling noise then, continued before giving him time to consider the number. "The Workers' Compensation checks you are receiving now fall under the category of temporary disability. It has to be determined by the caseworker and then by a judge at a hearing whether you are permanently or temporarily disabled."

Al gave another sarcastic sound of disgust. "Maybe we should have these people over for dinner, and I can show them my eyes or what's left of them." He took a breath and then continued to vent as Elaine stood by and gave him his moment. "I nearly died and I'm still hurt. All the information is in the medical records. I don't understand this." Al shook his head in anger and felt the familiar pressure he thought he had left behind on the operating room table.

Elaine turned to Al and hoped he was finished. "It's procedure. We're dealing with the New Jersey Disability and Social Security Administration. From what Mr. Bayplaza told me, a set amount of money that is awarded to victims for each type of injury and the amount granted is based on what the   judge reads from the book. We have to schedule appointments with the doctors that are paid by Worker's Comp as soon as you're up for it."

Resignation resonated in Al's voice. "Whenever you want to schedule them, go ahead."

Elaine looked sympathetically over at her husband. "The doctors we have to see are in Newark, Irvington, and The Oranges.

(125)

You have to see a doctor for your eyes, a psychiatrist, and a social worker. The state just wants a body to confirm that you are who you say you are as a procedural formality."

Al pushed his bar stool walked over to the fridge. "I need a new body, not a brain. Why do I need to see a shrink?" He yanked open the door and felt for the orange juice container. At the last second, he remembered to feel for the paper clip Elaine had put on the top of the container.

Elaine stared solidly at the paperwork in front of her. "We have to start selling our rental properties. If we unload the three we have and cut our losses, we can get through this."

Al had carried the orange juice over to the counter, found the glass he used in the sink and slowly began to pour. "At some point didn't you tell me that we have to pay all the money back to Worker's Comp if we win a judgment? I already had a policy to cover us that would not have made us pay them back. We're getting screwed." He took a sip and Elaine let him continue talking. "Selling the houses makes sense. We're breaking even on the Amboy house anyway after we collect the rent, so maybe we should cash out our equity. That money plus our savings will carry us through the rest of the year. Call Lou. We can trust him." The mention of Lou, Al's real estate agent, revived his spirit. Lou had always been honest and led Al toward the best
deals for rental property to purchase.

Elaine looked over at the glass of orange juice sitting on the counter. "Why are you drinking that? The acid must still bother your lips." She reached in her purse for the lip balm sent home with Al and watched him reach into the drawer she kept the straws in. The little steps he was making were monumental in the recovery process.

"What's next?" He took a dramatically long drink through the straw.

"Let me give you more background on what Art said in our meeting. More than one company will be involved in our lawsuit. He needs more information that only you can give him in

(126)

order to determine who those companies are. We have to claim the accident is 100% their fault."

Al did not stop drawing on a long sip of the orange juice until he was ready to speak. "No kidding."

"It's not personal, Hon." Al heard a professional tone or maybe it was resignation in her voice. "This is going to be about money and precedent, not about who is right. These companies are not going to want a lost case on their balance sheets. It makes them vulnerable to future lawsuits. A&K needs to make a claim that you are 51% responsible for your accident." Now it was Elaine's turn to gather her resilience before continuing. "Worker's Comp operates on percentages too and will be trying to prove that you were responsible for the accident."

Al began to shift immediately. "Sorry for all the moving around. My skin is bothering me more now that my head doesn't hurt so much." He squirmed around in his seat. "I wish I could shed my skin like a snake and start fresh."

Elaine looked over at Al, hesitated, and then pulled another paper out of her folder. "Let's get through this questionnaire from the lawyer as quickly as we can. Do you remember any of the manufacturers of the clothing you were wearing at the time of the accident?"

Al made another low whistling noise as his mind's eye went back to visualize the order forms that had passed over his desk. "BBLvd comes to mind first. BBLvd made the boots."

He brought his hand up to his chin and rubbed gently, barely touching the healing skin. This old habit he had clung to since High School always indicated to anyone around him that he was working through a difficult but solvable problem. Today, however, it offered him a painful reminder of the accident and the continuing aftermath.

"What about the equipment those three clowns pulled together? The lawyer can start with those manufacturers too." Al vented and felt the ironic comfort of tension release from his shoulders, head, and back. "I can't believe we can't go after those characters that created this mess. Charlie and the other two should be held for negligence." He shook his head slowly. "I understand the law but it doesn't make logical sense. If I went after those three I wouldn't be suing the company I would be suing their neglect of duty and ignorance of regulations."

"We need to do the best we can." Methodically, Elaine helped Al revisit the gruesome day, one failure at a time. "Didn't you tell me the safety shower head chain broke in your hand?"

"Yes." The feelings of desperation, potential relief, despair and panic of that day revisited themselves as he felt the chain hanging limply in his hand. "A&K should have had the shower inspected. We'll have to get inside the plant or obtain the records to check on the manufacturer. It was out of date and installed sometime in the 1950s." A new sense of purpose filled Al as anger rose inside him. "Check further into BBLvd as the mother company to Dlubthous, the clothing manufacturer. Look into Eunvea, Kao&Kao, and Nurradec. The last three I have to connect the dots to the products, but I've seen the names on orders."

Elaine raised her eyebrows and looked over the top of her glasses. "How do you know all this?"

"Who do you think signed the requisition orders? Who do you think was after the company brass to restructure the plant, reorganize the inventory and bring it into the 1970s?" Al felt the pervasive itching of his healing wounds become intolerable from sitting.

"The lawyer will be thrilled." She watched rub his chin. "This case will be on a contingency basis."

"I figured as much." Al felt the last of the afternoon sun make its way down the top of the window frame and touch his cheeks. The warmth felt good on his healing skin. He wondered how his new body would tolerate New Jersey winters. "Let me do some of the legwork with A&K. The company may want to appear cooperative and if not, I'll turn it over to Mr. Bayplaza." Al thought how good it felt to have a project that acted as a distraction from the constant discomfort he felt.

Elaine looked over at the man she was still in love with and cried inwardly at the pain he had suffered. "I think we're right in the approach we're taking. I'm betting the company will be cooperative since this is just the cost of doing business for them."

"All about business." Al placed the palms of his hands on his head.

The events of the accident replayed as he and Elaine completed the questionnaire. As he sat listening to her fold the paperwork and seal the envelope, he had an epiphany.

"Sweetheart?"

She looked at him cautiously. "Yes?"

He folded his hands calmly in front of him. "I never realized that until now, that I never have nightmares about that day. The only dreams I have are memories before the accident with you and the family when I could see you clearly. I see colors, I see life, but I don't see or relive the horrors or pain I went through. I never have dreams of escaping it either."

As Elaine sat quietly listening to her husband, one phrase came to her mind unexpressed to him. *Acceptance without resignation.*

Chapter X: Coping

Al began to take equal management of the finances and decisions concerning his medical care despite the discomfort and pain that continued to plague him. He spoke on the phone with the lawyer handling their legal case, Mr. Bayplaza, and at his request made appointments with the disability doctors. He asked Al to make the appointments for as early in the New Year as permitted by the doctor's schedules and Al's recuperation.

Al felt he was regaining some amount of control over his life when Christmas Eve arrived. He remembered Albert's first Christmas last year and how excited he and Elaine had been. Albert had been too small to understand the holiday then, but this year the toddler's face would be animated by the bright paper and pretty tree even if he still didn't fully understand who Santa was. Al felt himself drawn into the stark changes that had befallen them.

I may hear his voice, but I'll never see the look on his face. It will always be like this now. It's like sitting on the bench for the big game. I'll have to picture in my mind how everything looks as I participate at a distance.

"Al?" Elaine called to him from the other room.

He lifted his head wordlessly from where he sat on the edge of the bed. *I'm still in pain and discomfort. She knows I can't sit still for long, so I'll tell her the burns are bothering me more today because of anxiety. I don't want to do this. Everyone will remember last Christmas when I was whole. Besides, I'm itchy, sore, raw, and my headaches are back.*

Elaine prompted a response from him. "I don't want to be late. Are you ready?" She sat on the floor of the living room changing Albert one last time before leaving for the Christmas Eve party at her mom's house. She stood him on his feet as he grabbed at her necklace. "You like that? Daddy gave that to Mommy last year for Christmas." She smiled at the memory and at all the memories the future held. Joyful thoughts filled her mind. *My husband is alive. Our family is together for Christmas instead of visiting a grave and having masses said for him.*

Al wandered into the living room and purposely banged into the coffee table. "You know, I think maybe I'll hang here. My head is bothering me, and I could use time by myself. Do you mind?"

Looking up at him, her smile faded. "Yes, I do. The doctor said these day trips would be fine and this will only be for an hour with my family, yours and a couple of neighbors." She picked up Albert. "These are the people that love you and are happy you're alive. You can handle that." She turned and walked out of the room. "I'll meet you at the door."

Al heard her moving away from him and knew his efforts to avoid going to the party were futile. *I might as well get this over with.* He walked across the living room stealthily without the use of his cane. He reached the breakfast bar and found the cane propped on a bar stool with his coat draped across the back. He gingerly slipped his arms through the holes, still aware of the extra weight the clothing added on his healing skin. He felt how his shirt and pants hung on his frame. *I must look like a skeleton. I took a shower but my greasy hair is going to make me look like a slob.*

Feeling guilty about her tone with him, Elaine thought she would offer a compromise. "Al, do you want a Valium before we leave?"

"No. I'll rely on rum." He grabbed his cane.

(131)

"You're not supposed to have any alcohol with the medication you're on." Elaine stood with Albert in her arms.

"I realize that, Sweetheart. Please, let's just go." Albert began to fuss and Al's cynicism hit a wall. *Oh yeah, this is going to be great.* He attempted to calm Albert and lighten his own mood. "Santa's coming tonight. Remember?" Albert, still not completely aware of what Santa meant, fussed louder. Al climbed into his obligatory passenger seat and decided to go the extra mile and to stop thinking of only himself. "Honey, we'll have a good time tonight. I promise."

Upon arrival at the party, Al and Elaine were immediately greeted with overwhelming attention by well, meaning friends and family. Ronnie lifted Albert out of Elaine's arms to both the delight of himself and his parents. Al negotiated his way through the jovial group, desperately trying to distinguish voices. He managed to have Susan, a neighbor of his in-laws, take him over to Mr. Hinds at the bar for a 'soda'.

The cooperative woman was eager to get back to the food buffet. "Larry, give this young man a drink. If anyone deserves to celebrate, it's him."

Mr. Hinds smiled. "I agree. Susan, Helen made something special for you on the dessert tray."

Al leaned across the bar. "Dad, one shot of rum shouldn't be a problem with my medication. What do you say?"

Mr. Hinds looked sideways at Al as he shook a drink. "Are you sure it's safe?"

A man who Al didn't know walked up as the two were deciding Al's fate. "If any man in this room deserves a drink, this guy does. Thank God you're here with us. Merry Christmas, Al." He grabbed a beer off the counter and nodded at Mr. Hinds.

Mr. Hinds smiled. "That's two for two." He poured a small glass of rum and coke and pushed it to Al's hand. "Keep your mouth shut." He watched his son-in-law drain the glass. "You want another one to nurse?"

Al let the effects of the first drink wash over him. After three months, his lowered tolerance level allowed for a quick rush of the rum's generosity. "Yes, please."

Mr. Hinds poured the liquid into the glass in front of Al. "Sip this one. It's the last."

Al felt for the chair he knew would be next to the bar, sat down and waited for the night to be over. Throughout the evening neighbors and relatives continued to come up to him, wish him a Merry Christmas and say how good he looked. After hearing this over four times, the cynicism from earlier resurfaced.

What a crock. I probably look like a skeleton with a bad, peeling sunburn.

Eventually, he got up from the chair, stood next to it and waited for his father-in-law to notice him and come back to the bar. With two drinks already numbing the effects of the night and his physical discomfort, he figured what harm would one more do.

The older man had been watching Al from across the room and walked over and looked at Al's empty glass. "You can't think I'm going to fill that."

"Gimme a break, Dad." Al gripped the bar tightly.

"You'll put yourself into a coma." Mr. Hinds walked behind the bar and reached for the soda.

"I'll be fine. Just something to nurse. Please." He heard his father-in-law crack open the soda and place ice cubes in the glass in front of him. "Thanks, Dad."

"Don't tell your wife who helped you out. I'll hear about this for years." He poured a quick squirt of rum into the soda. "Only half a shot. You're cut off."

"Good enough." Al felt for the chair and slid into it.

The party concluded, and Al left without a memory of the drive home or finding his way to the master bedroom. Unable to blame the loss entirely on the combination of rum and the medications he was prescribed, he knew the emotional state he found himself in this Christmas season was symptomatic of the life-changing circumstances his family was enduring. He awoke the next morning to a miserable headache from the rum.

I wish I could spend the day in bed. How can I fake excitement and gratitude today?

(133)

Elaine had already been awakened by Albert, but held off bringing him to the tree until she heard Al stirring. She peeked into the doorway. "Merry Christmas." Elaine fought to control the squirming baby, who had been whining for his breakfast since his diaper change.

Al sat up slowly and moved into the sitting position at the edge of the bed. "It sounds like someone is ready to see what Santa left for him." He gingerly stood up as he tried desperately not to pitch forward. "I'll be right out." He began to make his way to the bathroom while Elaine continued to stand in the doorway with Albert.

I don't remember much about last night but she doesn't sound annoyed.

Al came out of the bathroom and the family made their way together to the Christmas tree. "Al, if you don't want to go to Fenna's for dinner I'll understand and be grateful. I don't want to rush around today. After Albert wakes up from his nap, maybe we'll go over for dessert." Elaine deposited the baby on the carpet and watched him squeal with delight as the tree and the presents came into view. "We'll blame our absence on you. You owe me one after last night."

The pretense was over. "How bad was I?"

Elaine laughed lightly. "Not terrible, I just need an excuse to relax at home." She sat next to Albert on the floor where he was transfixed by his new toddler size play restaurant. "Al, this is a riot. He keeps trying to eat the life-size fries that came with it."

Al felt a tightness in his stomach and talked quickly to get past it. "What's he playing with?"

Elaine realized her lapse. "I'm sorry. He's playing with the toy restaurant Santa brought. This thing is a really good replica that even includes life-size food." Elaine worked to pull the plastic food out of his mouth for the third time. "I don't think he's going to take a nap without a fight today."

Al laughed and imagined the sight of his son in front of the tree surrounded by toys. "He may not completely understand Christmas, but he knows a good thing when he sees it." The subtle

(134)

pounding in his head began to grow.

Elaine grabbed the plastic food. "Let me get him some fruit. Do you want me to make you something, Al?"

"You stay with him. I'll get the food." He walked to the kitchen avoiding any obstacles. What can I make you?"

"Al, I love you, but thanks anyway. I haven't eaten your cooking since the first week we were married. Just bring the fruit pieces for the little guy."

Laughing, Al reached on the counter for his radio. He pressed a button and Christmas music filled the room courtesy of the local station blending with the joyful noises of Albert tearing the paper off his presents as he squealed.

Al stood at the counter and lifted his head toward the happy noises. "Merry Christmas, Sweetheart. I'm glad to be here."

Chapter XI: Regaining Momentum

The melancholy Al experienced Christmas Eve grew steadily worse in January and mirrored the dreariness of the New Jersey winter that was cold but produced no snow. Depression had begun to take hold of him as the cold weather bothered his healing skin. He found himself wearing an extra sweater or carrying a throw blanket wrapped around his shoulders like an old man.

One day, as he crossed the living room to answer the phone, he walked into the wall. "Dammit!" He punched the wall and ripped off the picture that hung to the left of where he stood.

Albert, playing on the other side of the living room, burst into tears and Al yelled over the scared toddler. "Elaine! Could you get the phone?" He stumbled back to the couch ignoring Albert and gripped the hand that had done the damage to the wall.

After answering the phone call in the master bedroom, Elaine rushed to her son. "That was the furnace man. He'll be here in thirty minutes." She picked up the still whimpering baby and looked at Al's hand and his miserable expression. "Get yourself together." This was not Al's first outburst in the New Year and her tolerance was growing thin.

Al laughed derisively. "Are you kidding me?"

In disgust, Elaine walked back toward the bedroom with Albert in arms. "No, I'm not kidding."

Al talked to her back. "You want me to get it together for the furnace guy?"

Elaine stopped in mid-step. "No. I want you to get it together for me. At least change your clothes if you're not taking a shower."

Al rose from where he had been sitting for over an hour and grabbed at his sweatpants. Having lost interest in food and not eaten anything substantial in three weeks, his weight hovered somewhere around 135 pounds. He dressed like a slob and showered intermittently. His stubborn nature, developed since he was a kid, mixed today with self-pity.

If she expects me to clean up for the furnace man, she can forget it.

He walked around the couch kicking a few toys out of his way as he went. Walking to the wall he had damaged, he immediately felt regret as he ran his hand over the hole and loose bits of plaster ran between his fingers.

I'll fix this tomorrow. It won't look pretty but whatever I miss, Dad can clean up after me.

He was moving into the kitchen to retrieve a pan and broom when the doorbell rang. "Elaine? You want me to get that?"

Al wandered over to the front door still kicking any obstacles out of his way. He opened the door and was greeted by Vic, the mechanic from the furnace company and a fishing buddy of Al's from last summer.

"Hi, Al. It's Vic from Rapid Response." Vic stood in shock at the appearance of his friend. He wriggled into the house without being offered entry.

Al felt a little unbalanced as he closed the door and turned around. "Hi, Vic. Thanks for coming over. We're still trying to put spit and gum on the old furnace."

Vic, who had been friends with both Al and Elaine, had not seen Al at the hospital or since he had been home. He whistled as he stood staring at the gaunt, blind man before him. "Man, you look terrible."

Already angry in general and annoyed at the progression of his day so far, Al couldn't believe the audacity of this man whose company he used to enjoy. "Thanks. Had a bit of a rough time these last few months, in case you haven't heard.

Not at all dissuaded by Al's demeanor, Vic plowed ahead. "I'm not talking about your injuries. When's the last time you ate? When will you be taking your next shower?"

It took Al a minute to recover from the brutal honesty of his friend. "Still trying to adjust."

Vic stood perfectly still in front of Al. "To what? Life as a hermit? Vic placed his toolbox down next to his right leg as he watched Al pull upward on his sweatpants and maneuver past him to the couch.

Reminded of the world outside the confines of his life, Al felt embarrassed in front of Vic. "I, I haven't felt like eating much. The medication I'm on kills my appetite."

Vic followed Al and stood in front of the couch staring at him incredulously. "What medication are you on that kills your appetite for two months? Elaine said you made it out of the hospital in six weeks." He rubbed his calloused hand over the morning stubble on his chin. "You sound strong. You get around the house without a nurse holding your hand." In exaggerated exasperation, Vic dropped his hands from his face and held his palms out in front of Al as if he could see them. "You have to eat. This is no good. I don't care whether you're feeling sorry for yourself since you've been home or what, but you have to eat. Period. You're not going to get through this otherwise."

Al shifted on the couch and almost slipped sideways out of his sweats as his T-shirt slid off his right shoulder. "I know. I'm still getting back to normal."

Vic shook his head. "You're doing nothing to get back to normal." Vic sat down on the red love seat across from the matching couch. "When I first started to deal with my brain tumor I lost interest in food. It was depression. I had to make myself be interested in getting out of bed in the morning."

Al's head snapped up to face directly at Vic's level. "Brain tumor? You sound fine. How can you work?"

Leaning back on the overstuffed cushions of the love seat, Vic interlocked his fingers behind his head. "It was operable. I'm still on medication, but I learned early that you have to eat to have the strength to fight." He considered the fact that the man before him could not see. "You're skin and bones." Vic continued. "It sure would be a shame to have fought so hard and to quit now."

Al straightened his back and placed both hands on his knees. "I'm no quitter."

Vic smiled at his friend. "Good. What do you want for breakfast?"

"Eggs or pancakes." Al didn't want to tell Vic that part of the reason he was losing interest in food was the fact that he relied on Elaine to do the cooking for him and the guilt of the added work for her bothered him. "I was around 168 before the accident and now I'm around 135." Al felt like he was confessing.

Vic made another low whistling sound. "That's no good. You've got yourself this far why slack off?" Vic rose off the comfortable couch and stood to look down at his friend. "You can justify your behavior any way you want. It doesn't matter. You have to eat to move forward in your recovery."

Al held his right hand out and secretly hoped Vic wouldn't shake it too hard. "I'll start trying."

Vic cut Al short. "That's not good enough. Start now. If you need motivation, listen to the voices of your son and wife."

Al was speechless as his friend stood before him. "You're right." Humility washed over him before he continued. "I have to get moving now."

Vic took Al's hand in both of his, shaking it firmly but gently. "Time for me to get moving too. That furnace won't fix itself."

Al never noticed before how large Vic's hands were. "I think Elaine made coffee earlier. Please help yourself."

Vic poured a mug for himself. "I have two jobs after you

today, if I can fit everyone in."

Al started to move from his place in front of the couch toward the kitchen. *God bless this guy.* "Do you want some of the breakfast I have?"

Vic smiled. "Nah. I already had mine." He walked to the back door. "I'm heading for the cellar." He paused at the door to watch Al confidently walk across the room without his cane.

"The next time I see you, you better be heavier."

Al smiled and waved in the direction of Vic's traveling voice. "Next time? If you fix it right, we won't have to call you again." The fresh conversation and banter energized Al.

Vic opened the back door and laughed. "That old furnace needs to be put to rest. You better say a prayer that I can get it breathing. How much spit and gum do you think I have in me?"

Al tried to remember the day he stopped caring about what he looked like. "Elaine? Do we have coffee cake?"

Elaine came out of the bedroom with a clinging Albert holding tightly to her neck. "Yes. It's on the counter." She continued into the kitchen watching Al break off a large piece of coffee cake with his hands. "What prompted this?"

Between bites, Al responded. "I'm hungry." He reached into the cupboard for a plate. "Do we have any leftovers?"

Albert spotted his toys and squirmed out of her arms. "I can make you a sandwich or heat up the chicken."

"A sandwich would be great after my shower." Al continued to eat heartily.

Elaine stood looking at Al with grateful eyes. "I don't know what Vic said to you but I owe him the world." She decided this was a good time to tell him something she had been avoiding. "The Blind Commission is stopping by tomorrow."

Al swallowed the last of the cake on his plate. "I get it. I need some help." He wiped his hands of the crumbs over what he thought was the sink but was actually the counter next to the sink. "I'll be out in a while for that sandwich." He walked out of the kitchen and stood next to the hole in the wall he created earlier. Turning toward his creation, he used his hands to feel the damage.

(140)

"Elaine, would you mind getting me a hammer from the junk drawer?"

She leaned over the breakfast bar. "Are you planning on making the hole bigger?"

Albert came over to see what his Dad was doing next. "Hi Dada."

"Hi, Pal. Daddy has to clean up the mess he made. Sorry I scared you." He reached down and touched Little Albert's head.

"Hi, Dada." Albert ran back to his toys.

"Here." She handed the hammer she rescued from under rubber bands in her kitchen junk drawer to his outstretched hand. "I can't wait to see what you do with it."

Al found the picture lying on the floor where it had fallen. Without a glass front, he knew at least he did not have to worry about shards. Running his hand along the wall he felt the nail where the picture had hung and pulled it out with ease.

A few taps later he had moved the nail above the damage he created and hung the picture and looked for approval. "Elaine?"

"I'm here." She had been staring from the kitchen entry.

"What do you think?" He asked proudly with his hands on his hips.

She didn't try to hold back her smile and knew Al would hear it in her voice. "I think I'd better look behind all the pictures in this house."

Chapter XII: Guidance

The next day Lee Peterson from the Blind Commission arrived to assist Al in his adjustment to living in the larger world without sight. Elaine opened the kitchen door and he entered the house in a confident manner.

"Good morning Elaine. Is Albert ready?" Lee stood in the area where Elaine had welcomed him and waited for direction or Al's voice.

Elaine glanced over his shoulder to a car in the driveway. "Is someone waiting for you? Please tell them to come in and have coffee."

Lee shook his head slowly. "My driver today is my brother-in-law and he usually likes to sit and read while I'm on appointments."

"Are you sure?" Elaine started to leave.

"Yes." Lee inclined his head toward the open air in front of him.

Al heard Elaine greeting his new coach and called from the living room. "Hi, Lee. Come on in. You can sit on the love seat. I'll be across from you on the sofa. Does that work?"

"Good morning, Albert. That'll be fine. Is there a coffee table where I can lay out the items we may need?" Swinging his cane adeptly, Lee followed Al voice when he responded.

"Yes.   My wife tells me you can teach me how to cook. That's going to be a real improvement since I could never cook before the accident." Al tried to start the visit off on a light tone."

Lee walked closer to Al's voice and then felt his cane hit something. He reached down, felt the loveseat and began to settle in. "Eventually we'll get to cooking, however, let's start with maneuvering inside your home. I'm sure you heard how I entered the house and found my own way over to you without your wife's assistance. That's what we want to achieve with you. I want you to feel confident in your ability to move in and outside the world of your comfort zone. You've had time over the last two months to find your way around your home, but let's throw in some obstacles." Lee reached into the bag he had carried over his shoulder and pulled out a folding cane.

Al wondered if the lesson he was enduring would continue to be bland, business-like and boring. "You can't imagine the toys I've already maneuvered around," Al remembered yesterday and was glad Lee couldn't see the hole in the wall covered with the picture. "My attitude has improved dramatically too."

Lee continued without responding. "You seem to have accepted your loss of sight and that's the first hurdle. People can be stuck for months convincing themselves that it will return or become angry and sullen."

Al decided to drop the pretense. "I'm angry, but what's done is done. I lost interest in eating for a brief time." Al waited for a reaction as he heard the man sort through the items he brought. "A friend helped get me back on track."

Lee considered the physical trauma Al had experienced. "Are you limited anyway in your mobility?"

Al began to wonder how he measured up to Lee's other clients. "No. My burns are still healing and that makes it hard to sit still. The scarring is both painful and itches at the same time."

"The eating sounds more emotional than residual physical problems from the accident. I'm going to assume you are ready to move forward." Lee offered this as a statement and not a question.

Al felt his back stiffen and unconsciously clenched and unclenched both fists. "Let's do this." He shifted on the sofa nervously. "I hate to throw you a curveball, but what my eye doctor is working towards is a corneal transplant. I may have my sight back, even if it is only temporary."

"I hope for your sake that happens, but my job is to teach you to adapt to the world without sight. You can't stay inside all the time. You are going to want to go outside with your boy and be active." Lee appealed to the love Al had for his son. "I asked Elaine about what your life was like before the accident, and she told me you were a very active man socially, athletically and in your professional life. That doesn't have to change. You are just going to have to accommodate the inconvenience of living without sight."

Al jumped on the chance to talk about something that interested him and would lighten the mood. "I used to play a lot of ball. Actually, any kind of sport. I miss that."

Lee kept with the main topic, not wanting the man in front of him to become melancholy over what was lost. "People without sight do things that people with sight consider amazing, but people without sight call it the day-to-day chores of being alive. We go through the same routines sighted people do, it just takes us longer." Lee picked up the cane he had laid next to him on the loveseat and reached high across the coffee table. "Today we will be working on walking. I'm handing you a cane I brought. Which hand do you prefer?"

"The right." Al waved his right hand in the air until he caught the cane. "Are you the guy I'm always going to work with?" He gripped the cane, started to stand up, felt it give way, and leaned back immediately.

Lee smiled at Al's remark as he reached for his own cane and stood. "You'll get used to my style of teaching. My goal is to teach you to be independent."

Al ran his hand down the cane he held, realizing it was not meant to hold any weight and only to be utilized as a navigation tool. "Why can't I use the cane from the hospital?"

Lee stepped sideways to find a clear space away from the sitting area. "You can use either one. I thought you might want to get used to the difference between a folding cane and one needed for physical support." He tapped his cane on the carpet for effect. "I won't be the only person to assist your reentry into the world. Bob Evirdedis will be stopping by your home this week as you begin to develop a network within the blind community." Lee let Al move away from the couch and absorb the information he gave him.

Al began to slowly swing the cane in front of him. "This is much lighter than the other one. I like it." Al had a flashback to the blind man from his college days, scared and swinging the cane he held like a weapon.

Lee stepped back to avoid being smacked in the shin. "We want to help you develop a slow swing side to side close to the ground. You don't need to tap in here. Tapping is for unfamiliar surfaces."

Al slowed his swing of the cane but still hit a toy left on the floor. "Why do I have to do this in here? I have the whole house mapped out in my head."

"It's better to whack into an object than trip and fall flat on your face." Lee heard Al give the toy a sidekick. "You can't go into the world swinging a cane all over the place. Practice the repetition where you're comfortable and safe until you get the motion down." Lee listened as Al's cane tapped another toy and Al swatted it out of the way. "How many times have you tripped over toys in the last month? You may want to use that around here unless you can trust your two-year-old to pick up his toys and not expect your wife to make the house a safe environment for you."

Al stood still, memories of the scared blind man in his head. "Look Lee, I want to walk down the street looking as normal as possible. I can't do that holding a cane."

"Then get a dog or be prepared to spend a lot of time bleeding." Lee turned to move toward the kitchen. "The cane will give you confidence. As you are trying to look normal, you will be carrying yourself in regular strides. You'll never slow down

(145)

until your cane hits something."

"I don't like it," Al stated.

"I don't care," Lee responded. "You're doing great and I want you to continue to do so. It's easy to get stuck utilizing some bad habits when you don't realize you've slowed yourself down." Lee found the doorway to the kitchen and stood away from Al. "The basic technique is to alternate your steps with the movement of the cane. It should always be in front of the foot that is about to take the step and then sweep it to the other side. Back and forth, tap, tap, tap. It will be second nature to you over time."

"That's the blind leading the blind. If we get out of this alive, we'll be lucky." Al heard Lee laugh at his second attempt to lighten the mood.

The two men continued the monotonous practice around the house for almost an hour until Lee felt Al was confident in the movement. "Try not to deviate from the pattern I taught you until you've gotten used to it in the house. One potential problem for individuals without sight is snow."

"You mean there's only one?" Al continued to walk as Lee spoke.

"I stand corrected. Even if it is only one inch on the ground, it changes the topography and makes it difficult to tell what type of surface we are navigating. You can dig a little with the cane, but to be honest, unless it is absolutely necessary to go out while snow is falling or before it has been cleared from sidewalks and driveways, I personally would prefer to stay inside."

Al moved toward the sound of Lee's voice from where he had made a turn near the kitchen. "I'll try to remember that. We haven't had any snow yet this year, so we are due." He stopped by the plate of cake Elaine left out for the men. "I never offered you anything to munch on. Elaine left pound cake. Would you like some?" Al smiled inwardly at the offering she left for the men. "My wife always has cake and coffee ready." The gratuity of food was a staple that Elaine had adopted from her mother.

Lee moved toward the sofa and the bag he had brought. "No, thank you. I'm going to lunch with my brother-in-law."

Al grabbed a thick slice and ate as he walked, talking around his mouthfuls. "I can't wait to get outside and walk on the gravel driveway. Our street is asphalt so I should have no problem taking walks around the neighborhood." The possibility of more independence energized him.

Lee prepared to leave. "The first couple of times it would be a good idea to take your wife with you." He didn't want to diminish Al's positive attitude, but he also didn't want this new student to lose touch with the reality of his world.

"I got it. Independence without complete freedom." His acknowledgment spoke volumes.

Lee zipped up his bag and turned to walk toward the door. "Living without sight involves the entire family." He reached for his cane. "You've got a long road ahead of you, but you can manage. I've worked with people that couldn't and it took years of struggle to move past the bitterness of a sudden loss of sight."

Al swallowed another mouthful of cake and then spoke. "What other choice do I have?"

Lee talked over his shoulder. "I think you already tried your other choice recently. You've chosen this now." Lee straightened and stood squarely before Al. "See you next week, same day."

Al heard the man move toward the door. "Will the lessons be this short?"

Lee reached the front door and smiled for himself guessing that Al could hear his encouragement in his voice. "No. You still have to meet with Bob and then we can move along. The lessons will get longer. You're a quick study. You'll do fine." He felt the door handle and called back. "Take it easy and practice. Practice, practice, practice."

"Thanks for your time." The door slammed shut behind Lee and Al heard Elaine come into the room.

"That was pretty quick. How did it go?" She stood a little wide-eyed.

Al moved back to the kitchen, not bothering to practice with the cane. "Good. He's a nice guy. A little dry, but a nice guy."

(147)

"Your personality will lighten the mood. When is the next session?" Elaine watched Al polish off the pound cake and smiled.

"Next week, same day and I assume the same time. I should have the whole neighborhood mapped out in my head by then." Al was thoughtful. "Do you know anything about the second guy the commission is sending this week?"

Elaine leaned on the breakfast bar across from Al. "The only information they gave me is that he is sighted and acts as your liaison with the Blind Commission. He is not a professional counselor, he is a facilitator to ensure you're getting everything you need from the program. You need to communicate and cooperate thoroughly with him. Don't hold back your thoughts."

Al nodded agreeably. "That seems straightforward enough. I'll give anything a try."

Bob Evirdedis, the sighted man working for the Blind Commission, visited three days later to discuss the assistance Al would be receiving and how he felt about it. The assurance and positive attitude Bob witnessed confirmed that Al was ready to integrate into society as a blind individual and needed the commission's help to learn navigation while he healed physically.

"Are we doing any lessons today?" Al was getting bored and either wanted to move forward with a lesson this day or spend time with his son.

"No. Today I wanted to check in with you in person to gauge where you were at in your recovery." He studied Al's response. "Did your wife explain my position within the agency?"

"Yes. I guess I thought we would be working today." Frustration was evident in Al's tone.

"I understand. Lee will be back next week and you will move forward with the inclusion of learning the Braille system." Bob looked up at Al as he wrote his summary of the meeting. "There are social groups for you and your wife to join."

Al shrugged his shoulders amicably. "That sounds appropriate. My wife has been through hell. It would be a good idea for her to be around others dealing with some of the same issues we are."

Bob looked at Al and privately acknowledged to himself how advanced his new client was in his recovery. The empathy Al expressed for the person and people closest to him spoke of his connection to the larger world. Confident in Al's ability at continued growth, Bob established a lesson schedule for Al that was going to introduce the Braille reading system. He held a phone conference with Lee after his initial meeting and instructed him to move the lessons forward expeditiously.

Al met Lee enthusiastically at the door the following week. "Thanks for coming. Guess I didn't scare you off."

Lee breezed past Al walking confidently with his cane by memory to the loveseat and began unpacking his bag immediately. "It's a pleasure working with you. You're a quick study. Not all my clients are as responsive as you. This is going to be a breeze."

Al followed behind Lee and had to admit he had to rush to keep up. "How do you move so quickly?"

Lee laughed lightly. "Once I've been somewhere, I commit the layout to memory. It comes second nature to me from years of practice."

Al sat down heavily on the sofa. "I'm ready for whatever you have planned this morning."

"Can you tell me how bad the scarring is on your hands?" He placed a book and a stack of cards, each of which was the size of an index card on the coffee table.

"The scarring on my hands is on the top. Why?" He shifted uncomfortably.

"Relax, today is your first Braille lesson." Lee felt the cards he had laid out.

Al shifted continuously against the cushions. "I'm not nervous, I'm tormented by the itchy healing burns. The dermatologist gave me a cream that's doing absolutely nothing." He took a long sip of the chamomile tea he had left on the coffee table that his mother recommended to relax him. "I think the dermatologist is a clown."

Lee had laid out the necessary teaching paraphernalia between them. "I'm sorry to hear that. Let's get started and maybe

(149)

the lesson will help take your mind off the itching." He picked up the first card. "In front of you on the coffee table are cards with large Braille print. You'll notice that I call it print." He slid the first card to Al's left. "Card one is to your left. Reach down and run your hand over the dots." Lee digressed from the lesson. "Braille was invented by Louis Braille during WWI for messages that the troops could read in the dark.

Al reached over and felt the index size card with large dots on it. "Are the dots always this big?"

"No. These are your introductory cards." He gave Al a minute to feel the print. "We will begin by using the larger cards for introduction and concept. You'll be feeling regular sized print before the end of the day."

Elaine came into the room. "Hi, Lee. Nice to see you."

Lee waved. "Hi, Elaine. Al's a pleasure to work with."

Elaine moved about the kitchen getting food for Albert. "Lee, would you like some tea or coffee? I could make breakfast if you're hungry?"

"Coffee would be great." Lee began to push a second card toward Al. "On the first card six dots which create the Braille cell. The raised dots are configured in two columns, three dots each. Starting from the top, the raised dots are numbered, one, two, three in the left column and four, five, and six in the right. That is the basic cell that you have to memorize because it is the building block for the alphabet." Lee reached across and brought Al's hand to where he wanted it on the card.

Al stopped shifting immediately. "I got it."

Elaine brought over the steaming cup of coffee. "Lee, here's your coffee in a heavy mug about six inches from your left hand.

"Thank you. What time is it at?" Lee very slowly began to move his left hand.

Elaine's voice reflected how puzzled she was by his question. "Excuse me?"

Lee turned his head away from Al and toward Elaine. "I'm Sorry. What I am asking for is the position of the mug if it was on the face of a clock. We haven't gotten to that lesson yet for Al. It's the easiest and the most practical for dining out or at home."

Elaine gave her best guess. "Oh. I would say nine o'clock." She smiled appreciatively. "Looks like I'm getting a lesson today also." She left the room quietly.

Lee found the mug and felt the inviting warmth of the ceramic. "Thank you." He enjoyed a long sip and returned it to the same place. "Your left hand will be an indicator of what line you are on."

As Al ran his finger over the dots, he projected ahead how he would utilize this methodology for labeling boxes, drawers in the bedroom and in the kitchen. "This is a good system. I can understand the practical need for it."

Encouraged, Lee pushed the second card he placed on the table closer to the first. "Move your hands to the next card I laid out for you to the right of the first. This card has smaller dot sizes. As you are feeling them, I want you to start thinking about the alphabet. For each letter of the alphabet, the Braille dots will be arranged in a specific order. For example, the letter A is represented by the dot in position #1 in the Braille cell. The letter B is represented by dots in #1 and #2 in the Braille cell." Lee continued until the entire alphabet was explained and then moved forward to numbers. "The first ten letters also represent numbers. The indicator between numbers and letters is what comes before the number which represents a number sign." Lee moved Al's finger over the dots making the sequence. "The indicator is the dots in position 3,4,5, and 6."

Al continued to feel the dots with his finger. "This will take time to learn. These days I have a lot of that."

"It's all rote, hard-core memorization." He lifted another card with even smaller dots off the top of his deck and pushed it next to the second. "This card has dots on in that are the size you will normally find in your readings."

Al moved his hand over and began to rub the tiny raised dots. "You've got to be kidding me. I can hardly find these."

Lee heard the intensity which Al applied to the card. "Try

(151)

not to pick at the raised dots. I use the cards with other students."
He tried to backtrack over his admonishment. "You'll get used to them, believe me."

Al continued almost digging at the raised dots. "I swear these dots are not raised off the card as high as the larger cards."

"That's correct. Let's go over the letter C." Lee started to redirect his student's thoughts.

In frustration, Al interrupted him. "Not yet. Let me get used to the feel of these. I won't have a problem with the concept of the arrangement or memorizing the letter, but feeling and identifying the set up that's going to be a challenge. Maybe I should soak my fingers in dish detergent first to soften them up."

Lee scoffed agreeably. "At least you have a sense of humor."

Al stopped feeling the dots. "Who's kidding?"

Lee lifted something from his bag. "I want to take some notes while you're studying the cards," Lee spoke into the tape recorder he brought and then turned back to Al. "Have you started marking your food in identifying manners?"

Al stopped running his fingers over the card he held. "Are you recording us?"

"No, taking notes for myself as reminders of what to say to Bob Evirdedis. My Braille writer is too big to carry around. I'll retype the report for him when I get back to my home office so we can keep track of your progress." Lee shut off the recorder. "You may prefer to have a Braille stylist. It's a small plastic instrument that slides and punches the holes for whatever you are writing. I don't have one with me today." He put the recorder back into his bag.

Al continued to run his fingers over the cards and attempt to memorize letters A to D. "Bob and you are both thorough."

"He'll want to know where you're at so that he can decide which field trips to take you on outside the walls of your home and which practical applications to start working on."

"I already take lots of field trips with my wife." Al didn't bother to contain his irritation at the suggestion of something that sounded like a Grade School expedition.

"Is she blind too? You need the experience of a person who trains those without sight to teach you. How are you going to learn to cross a road if Elaine is always with you? Your cane can hit the low stuff, but what about the obstacles that protrude into your walking space waist high? You have to adapt to the world as if you lived in it alone. You have to rely on your other senses." Lee finished and tried to gauge Al's response.

Al grudgingly accepted the reality Lee tried to make him face. "I'll find a way to adjust to the idea." He piled the Braille cards together and ran his fingers over the top card.

Lee smiled, "I told Bob you're an engineer. You're analytical and a quick study." Lee turned off his recorder and packed it into the bag. "You never told me how you are doing with food."

Al continued picking at the Braille dots on the top card of the stack he had made. "I put a paper clip on the OJ container and leave the milk without."

"Good. Let me offer a few suggestions. If the containers are different shapes, that works, but if not, tear the flap according to what the brand is. Different brand, different position of the tear. Paper clips can be knocked off. This identification is not only for your convenience, but for the respect of those you live with. Nobody wants to drink orange juice after someone else had his nose in it trying to determine what it was. Those of us living without sight can't live in the world as if we're alone."

"I mark my cereal with tape in different positions for my favorite to second favorite, etc. I'm pretty good with the microwave too. Greatest invention to come out of the 1960s. I marked the dial so I know where one minute is." Al kept going. "I can cook an egg or small cake in a minute. I started to make a game of it by seeing if I can eat the first egg before the second one is done. Can't imagine what my arteries look like."

Lee sat up straight. "That's excellent. How do you pour drinks for yourself?"

Al began to think he should teach blind students. "Over the

drain board or the sink."

Lee clasped his hands in front of himself and listened as Al moved the top card he picked at to the bottom and felt the dots on the next. "How about when you are out with your wife?"

"Hasn't come up yet. In my condition, I really haven't wanted to go out." Al shifted in the chair and thought briefly about Christmas Eve.

"I understand your social limitations right now. When you are feeling better and you are at a friend's house, ask for a bowl or a saucer to place under your cup or glass. If you want to add your own milk, tip your mug, placing the tip of your finger inside for measuring." Lee reached for his coffee and took a sip.

Al anticipated laundry would be the next subject discussed. "I wash my own clothes separately and I use safety pins positioned in seven different utilizing the face of a clock to categorize colors, work, dress, etc., on the inside of my clothing. My socks are pinned together the minute I pull them off my feet and are put in the wash that way. I feel the difference between pants, shirts, shorts and undershirts. I generally wear jeans, khaki pants, white T-shirts, and tan shorts, but I do have polo shirts, oxfords and a few colored T-shirts. I don't wear pajamas and I pin my underwear on the right side of the elastic to tell inside from out. My white undershirts are pinned on the right and jeans are pinned on the inside front pocket. I keep my oxford shirts hanging in the closet and pin them according to the color of the pattern. I never take any of the pins off, but if I lose them in the wash and I can't discern by touch what type of pants I'm holding, I have to ask my wife. To categorize storing my clothes, I have the drawers in my dresser sectioned off for my white, black and brown socks. To save time, I try to group my T-shirts with the pants I like so I'm not mismatched."

"I didn't know you were physically able to organize all this." Lee smiled. "You're way ahead of me."

Al shifted while he spoke. "I can't sleep all day even if I don't feel well. With this much time on my hands, I apply the basic principles of an engineer for all the aspects of living without sight. First, I identify the problem, second, I collect the data, third, I analyze the data, find solutions available, fourth, I analyze the solutions, and finally, I go with the best one. This might sound stupid to the average Joe Q Public, but for me, each problem I have to solve keeps my mind busy."

"You're doing better than I expected. You don't know how to quit. I believe what you went through at the beginning of this winter is behind you permanently." Lee sat back.

Al was thoughtful before he responded. "My High School guidance counselor who was supposed to help me with college told me not to bother and to 'get a job.' I got angry, worked harder at my High School classes, was accepted to the Newark College of Engineering and did very well in my undergraduate studies. I don't like anybody or any situation dictating what I can or cannot do." Al began to pick aggressively at the top Braille card.

"Would you like me to leave the cards with the normal size dots here for your practice?" He could hear Al scraping the cards.

"I don't know how many dots will be left if you leave the cards with me." Al felt a stack of five cards pushed toward him.

"I'll come by next Friday and see how you feel and then maybe we can proceed further into the alphabet. Keep them but try to be gentle." Outside a car horn beeped. "That's my driver. I told him that I was on a bit of a tight schedule today and to let me know after an hour had passed." Lee pulled his coat on, grabbed the cards he was not leaving with Al and shoved them into the bag. "You'll master the alphabet and then we can work on simple words, and eventually increase your speed at reading them." He began to move toward the door, his cane guiding him. "You're doing well. Remember, Braille is the only thing you do one handed when you are blind. You have ten eyes between your two hands, use them together for everything else. Anything outside the two-foot length of your arm requires you to move and creates the biggest day-to-day challenge of living without sight. To be blind is to be organized and you're off to a running start. A person without sight cannot spend two hours looking through laundry or attempt to function in the larger world with mismatched clothes or bad manners."

Al stood and followed Lee's retreating figure through the kitchen to the back door. "Thanks for your help."

"You're quite welcome. Take care. I'll see you next week." Lee reached for the door handle and let himself out.

Elaine emerged from the bedroom carrying Albert. "How was your session today?"

"I can utilize my engineering principles for skills to adapt to most things but not for Braille. I can't feel the dots. It's ridiculous." Al shook his head and laughed.

Elaine ran her hand across the card. "Wow, I had no idea the dots were this small."

Albert grabbed at the card and tore it slightly.

Al laughed when he heard the small tear. "That's pretty much the way I feel about them."

All three began to laugh. The sound filled the house.

Chapter XIII: Reprieve

Al continued to work on his cane skills as the discomfort from his healing burn tissue grew. At one point the skin appeared translucent and baby soft after Al had left the hospital debridement procedures behind him. Scarring developed as the extreme pain decreased and the torturous itching from the healing tissue increased. The one proven method to counter the itching and attempt to minimize the consequential scarring was to fool the body into thinking it was already finished with healing the damaged tissue by the utilization of a pressure garment. This pressure garment was worn by the affected individual for an indefinite period of time almost immediately after an injury. Unfortunately, throughout the winter of 1975, Al was not made aware of the device needed and he suffered accordingly. The combination of the itching, the scarring, and increased headaches from the rebuilding eye pressure grew together at an alarming rate.

The extreme head pain he had experienced at the beginning of December was replaced with a constant feeling of strong pressure and sporadic intense migraines. During the February 8th visit to Dr. Westmont's office, the doctor thought the eye could perforate at any time.

"Mrs. Plevier, you need to drive him to Manhattan Eye and Ear hospital now. I'll call ahead and have Dr. Leesville meet you. I had already briefed him on Al's case, but Al needs a corneal plug today." He turned back to Al sitting in the exam chair. "Al, you told me the headaches were normal. What I am seeing can only be accompanied by the same excruciating pain you suffered at Thanksgiving."

Al held his head in his hands as he spoke. "What's normal? Sometimes it hurts like hell. I thought that's what the drugs were for until another surgery was scheduled."

Dr. Westmont turned back to look into Elaine's frightened eyes. "I can have him transported by ambulance if you would prefer."

Elaine rose from her chair and moved to stand next to the examination chair where Al sat in misery. "I'm fine as long as it's safe for him."

Elaine had never driven in Manhattan. She and Al had grown up in Paterson which had public transportation. After they were married, Al did most of the driving. Gone now were the weekends the family would get into the car without a specific destination, drive as fast as Elaine would tolerate and eventually arrive back home. Today Al had no time to think about the joy he used to feel behind the wheel of any car and Elaine did not have time to think about her dread and nonexperience navigating Manhattan streets. Today they found themselves again in survival mode.

Dr. Westmont and his nurse ushered Al into the elevator while Elaine rushed to retrieve the car and pull it to the front of the building where she met Al standing next to the nurse. He fell asleep almost immediately from the codeine he had been given at the office, leaving Elaine to focus on the journey. Traveling through the Lincoln Tunnel she was shocked at how easily she navigated across Manhattan then uptown to the 64th Street address. At the Emergency Room entrance of Manhattan Eye and Ear, she left Al in the car while she found a nurse with a wheelchair.

"You made better time than we expected, Mrs. Plevier. Dr.

Westmont's office called us."

Elaine bent down to kiss Al good-bye without commenting on the travel time. "I love you. I'm going to park the car, but I'll be back in the hospital before the procedure is over."

Al lifted his head from its place in his hands and called over his shoulder to her. "I love you too." He tried to speak above the serenading screams and pleas of the young children waiting to be triaged that greeted him through the opened doors. "Somebody help those poor kids. Was there a bus crash or something?"

The nurse waited until the chair was farther away from the tortured sounds of the children to respond. "No, Mr. Plevier. Unfortunately, this is not an uncommon day for us here."

"Did we enter through the Pediatric Ward?" Al dropped his head back into his hands.

The middle, aged nurse breathed out heavily as she pushed him. "No. We have a lot of children that come here either for emergency care or through the ER for their routine visits."

Thinking outside of his own misery, Al's heart broke for the children. "That has to be one of the worst sounds I've ever heard."

Elaine tried to watch Al until the wheelchair turned the corner, but she too was suddenly aware of the suffering children in the waiting area. The pitiful sounds broke her heart as she met the gaze of one mother who smiled weakly at her. Elaine smiled back sadly before running out to move the car.

The cries of the children had not lessened when she returned through the public entrance by the phone booths. The additional distance lowered the volume of the cries that met her ears, but not their urgency. She sifted through the bottom of her purse for a dime, finally gave up, picked up the receiver and asked the operator to make a collect call from Elaine.

Mrs. Hinds answered. "Hi, Hon. What's wrong? I thought the visit would only be for an hour." Elaine's Mom held the phone with one hand and helped Albert color with the other.

"Mom, we're at Manhattan Eye and Ear Hospital in The City." Elaine clenched the stiff receiver line and felt herself catch her breath.

"What happened?" Mrs. Hinds continued to watch Albert scribble over the large coloring book his grandpa had bought him.

"Dr. Westmont felt the eye might perforate at any moment. The glaucoma is continuing to build pressure." The smell of the hospital pervaded Elaine's senses and she wrinkled her nose. A wave of familiarity and nausea washed over her as their latest emergency and the stress of the anticipated drive home bore down.

"Do you want Dad to drive into the city and sit with you?" Mrs. Hinds looked out at the afternoon winter sky.

"No, I'm nervous about driving back out of the city at night, but I have to start getting used to this. We'll be making more trips to this hospital and I don't want to keep bothering you." Elaine squeezed her eyes shut and held the receiver cord with her free hand. "The traffic won't be bad by the time I leave."

"You know we're happy to help. If you really are determined to drive home alone tonight, call us before you leave." Mrs. Hinds returned to watching Albert and found herself in a struggle of wills as the little boy protested while she pulled a crayon away from his mouth.

"Is Albert fussing?" Elaine felt very tired.

"He's fine. He's just not interested in his dinner." She wiped the toddler's mouth and unclasped the high chair tray. "Have you eaten?"

"No. I'll run to the cafeteria. I want to make sure I'm there when Al comes out of recovery." She opened her eyes and stared at the fluorescent bulbs overhead.

Mrs. Hinds unbuckled Albert and lifted him to the floor and his freedom. "Don't forget to call later before you leave."

"I won't. Thanks, Mom." Elaine hung up the phone and started towards the cafeteria.

When she returned to the waiting area a nurse in the Emergency Room directed her to the seventh floor where Dr. Leesville was waiting. She proceeded upstairs without any indication from the nurse as to Al's condition or what to expect. She was met on the on the seventh floor by a tall, thin man with a substantial mane of salt and pepper hair.

Elaine approached him quickly. "Excuse me, are you Dr. Leesville?"

Dr. Leesville closed the chart he was writing in and turned his attention to the woman in front of him. "Yes. You must be Mrs. Plevier." He extended his hand and gently accepted hers. "Albert is in recovery. He did very well. We placed the corneal plug in his left eye. This will prevent the cornea from perforating and being susceptible to infection." He looked for recognition on her face and when he did not find any, he continued with an explanation. "A corneal plug is a donor cornea stitched over the entire cornea of his left eye. We enlarged it so that it will not perforate. The chemical in the initial injury had begun to eat the cornea. The closest similarity I can offer is that of a blowout patch on a tire. The transplant is a temporary fix. The surgery went very well, but he'll need to remain in the hospital for another week."

"Can I see him?" Elaine could think of nothing except being next to her husband.

Dr. Leesville looked down into Elaine's weary face with compassion. "Absolutely, but don't expect too much. He is still coming out of the anesthesia."

She crossed her thin arms over her upper body and realized how pleading her gesture made her appear. "I just want to look at him. If he knows I'm there, then the ordeal is manageable for us."

Moved by the love Elaine and Al shared, Dr. Leesville picked up the chart he had been writing on and smiled warmly at her. "Follow me."

Elaine was led down a hallway into a recovery area and asked to put on a mask and gown. Three other patients were in the room with Al. She stared at him and spoke to Dr. Leesville. "When will Al be moved into a semi-private room?"

Dr. Leesville covered his mouth while he yawned widely. "I apologize, but I've been on call and had two emergencies early this morning. Albert can be moved to a semi-private room late tomorrow if he is still progressing, but if not, we will want to keep him in ICU for observation." Dr. Leesville gazed at his patient in the hospital bed motionless. "I don't think we have anything to worry about. He is doing well and there is hope for saving the left eye. He still may be eligible for a corneal transplant if his progress continues."

Elaine walked across the white room through subdued artificial lighting. Natural light from outside streamed in through large double hung windows toward her husband's bed. She leaned down close to his ear.

"Al, I'm here and you are doing great. I'm going to go home in a little while, but I'll be back early tomorrow after I get the baby settled." Elaine touched Al's hand and turned to walk out of the room.

The all too familiar routine of hospital stays had reestablished itself and she found herself completing the mental checklist of the logistics and questions she had to ask the doctor in charge. "Dr. Leesville, you look as tired as I feel."

Dr. Leesville smiled and rubbed his eyes behind his glasses. "I'm used to the hours, but I don't think my family ever will be. I'll be leaving the hospital in two hours but I will be on call. The doctor on floor duty has been briefed on your husband's case."

She gazed briefly at the windows as she spoke. "Doctor, be honest with me, please. Will Al ever have a chance to regain his sight or is he going through all this misery that could be avoided if he had both his eyes removed?" Elaine turned to stare directly into the doctor's face hoping that she could see beyond his professional demeanor.

Dr. Leesville did not hesitate to answer. "I believe there is a chance. Medicine is making extraordinary advances and with Albert's age and the status of his health prior to the accident, he makes a perfect candidate for the trial medications he has been on. I want to focus on a corneal transplant after he regains the weight he lost and the other injuries from the accident are further along in the healing process."

Elaine closed her eyes tightly and reopened them slowly as

(162)

she spoke. "Al will always want to keep trying if there is any chance at all. I won't try to talk him out of that." She looked down at the floor and then back into the face of the man in charge of the possibility of Al ever seeing his family again. "I should start back home. Driving in The City is not something I enjoy."

The doctor looked at her with compassion. "Write down any questions you may think of tonight, and we can go over them when Albert becomes fully conscious." Dr. Leesville smiled weakly at Elaine, touched her shoulder lightly and then turned to walk away.

Elaine left Al's room and then stopped briefly at the exit to phone her parents before completing the uneventful ride from Manhattan to Wayne.

The next morning, she repeated the cycle and breathed deeply as she pulled into the familiar parking garage from yesterday. As she was about to enter the hospital, the sound of a single engine plane over the noise of the city traffic caught her attention. She looked up and was immediately brought back to Al's interest in flying.

Last year he had purchased plans for an airplane kit and was determined to put it together over the winter and fly it this spring. She closed her eyes tightly, remembering for the first time since last summer that the plans still sat in the far corner of the garage in boxes, but the kit had not been ordered yet. The private flying lessons he had taken were compensation for not qualifying for the Air Force pilot program, a secret dream he had always had. Elaine had not fought him on flying an experimental aircraft, but worried incessantly about the safety of the single-seat, propeller plane. She shook her head at the irony as she continued to walk into the hospital.

Al was fully awake and sitting up when she came into his room. "Hi, Al. How are you feeling?"

He turned his head toward her voice. "Hi, Sweetheart." He lifted his left hand, hoping she would take it and was not disappointed.

"I just arrived. Did Dr. Leesville come to see you?" Elaine

dropped a kiss lightly on his cheek.

"He was in for a few minutes." Al relaxed. "I feel terrible. How do I look?" He gave her a weak smile.

Elaine looked grimly at Al. "About as good as you feel. Did he tell you that you have to stay for a week?"

"Yes. The narcotics are helping with the burns also. I need this reprieve. Who's watching Albert?" He pictured a little hand pulling his dad toward whatever toy was near.

"Your mom took a day off work. I think the two of them need some grandma time." She let go of his hand to pull a chair next to the bed. "What do you want me to do for you? Maybe I can ask if a radio is allowed." She sat down and reached up for his hand.

"Don't worry about it. I really don't think I could stand the background noise. I want to rest. Maybe you should stay home tomorrow. I know the driving must be killing you." Al relaxed his head.

"Not seeing you would kill me." Elaine gripped Al's hand tighter."

Al turned his head back. "Elaine, Dr. Leesville believes there is a chance I can get my sight back even if it's only temporary."

"I know. He spoke to me about it last night." Elaine was glad he couldn't see her face. "If you think the chance is worth the pain and misery you have to go through, then I support you."

"Worth it? Any chance I have of looking at you or our son is worth it. Forget about getting on with the business of life, I want to see you." Al felt weak from the sudden outburst of emotion.

Elaine closed her eyes as she spoke to her husband. "You know I will support whatever you decide. Get some rest. I'll be here until early afternoon."

He gathered up some energy. "Elaine?"

"Yes?" She stopped getting up from the chair.

"Could you pick out a pair of glasses for me? Something dark that people can't see into and large enough to cover my eyes completely, without looking like Jackie O." Al scratched his chest.

"Make sure the glasses are stylish and not made for a blind person."

"Maybe I should hire a designer to help me out." She got up to leave.

"I was lying here remembering that dinner we went to at your colleague's house last summer. The blind woman got up to use the bathroom one of the other couples said she should get glasses because of how disgusting her eyes looked." Al turned his head toward Elaine and squeezed the hand he still held. "I don't want to be viewed as somebody who doesn't care about my appearance. I'll be bandaged with the goggles for a little while longer, but in the future, there's no reason for my family to be embarrassed by the stuff I can control."

She stood and leaned over to kiss his healed lips. "Whatever you want. I have to find Dr. Leesville. I'll be back after I talk to him." She gave his hand one last squeeze and walked out of the room.

Elaine spent the next hour waiting for Dr. Leesville in the family area. While she sat in the crowded room, she watched the number of children that came in. Children of all ages arrived accompanied by worried parents. The miniature humans sat in the waiting room chairs gripping their favorite toys and continuously asking how much longer.

Dr. Leesville approached Elaine as she was deep in thought watching a little boy trying to find the toy he had rolled out of reach. "Good Morning, Mrs. Plevier."

"Hi, Dr. Leesville." She absently looked at her watch. "It's almost afternoon."

"My apologies. I lose track of time when we get busy. Do you want to go to my office?" He looked at the crowded room.

"No, this is fine. It helps me keep a clear perspective on our own circumstances." Noticing the parent of the child with the truck was busy filling out paperwork, she reached down and rolled the little match box truck to the child. He felt the car and smiled broadly.

The doctor took the seat next to Elaine. "Tomorrow Albert

will feel complete relief from the cessation of the building fluid. Without an intense headache, he'll be able to move forward with your lives while we continue working on his recuperation. The eventual goal, after he is stronger, is to prepare him for a corneal transplant."

She nodded in agreement. "That's what Al wants. I believe the long, term goal to see gives him additional motivation to listen to his doctors and do what he is told." Elaine stared at the doctor.

He looked intently into Elaine's face. "The most important thing now is that he gains weight. Even if a cornea match became available tomorrow, we could not perform the procedure. The time is too close to the initial injury. Healing needs to take place in his eyes and his body."

Elaine glanced around the room at the little boy. "I understand." Acceptance that Al had a long recovery regardless of the potential for his sight to return was not a burden. She wanted him to recover so that their little boy would have a father to love. "I'm grateful to you for taking away the pain and continuing to salvage his eyes. Offering him potential that he might see our son helps him cope day to day. Having him home and knowing he is getting stronger, helps me cope. There a light at the end of the tunnel for both of us."

Chapter XIV:
Enlightenment and Human Nature

By the end of March, the appearance of Al's healing burn injuries was slow but substantial. The facial wounds had become forty percent healed within the first six weeks of the hospital stay, but the burns on his torso, arms, hands, and feet from the sodium hydroxide were, six months after the accident, a source of increasing discomfort. Itching, soreness, and sensitivity to cold continued from the extra fluid buildup that caused scar tissue. The discomfort was constant and seemed to be increasing. Al and Elaine had already sought the medical advice of a dermatologist, outside the Overlook hospital network. He had been chosen out of the phone book and after a brief exam, in which he did not ask Al to take off his shirt, he explained that the itchiness he felt was caused from the boredom of Al's expulsion from the workforce. According to this dermatologist, he was spending too much time thinking about his healing body. He sent Al home with a prescription for an ointment which was ineffective.

(167)

Immediately after returning home from the latest dermatologist follow up appointment, Al phoned his cousin Francine, who was a nurse. "I need a dermatologist who knows what he's doing. There has to be relief besides Valium." Al moved around on the chair trying to find relief rubbing against the back.

Francine opened the medical network address book she kept at her desk. "A plastic surgeon named Dr. Grove specializes in burn victims and has had a lot of success. I haven't talked to him in a while, but you can call his office this afternoon and for the first available appointment."

Al's misplaced irritation at his cousin grew. "Why didn't you give me this guy's number sooner?"

"I thought you were working within Overlook's network." She knew everything her cousin had been through and tried to be understanding. "Your injuries are beyond the scope of an ordinary dermatologist. You have to continue with specialists in each of your areas of need." Francine had the number in her Rolodex and recited it. "How are you writing this down?"

"Paper and pencil." He had a piece of paper in front of him and a ruler to write in the manner Lee Peterson had taught him. He rubbed his back as Francine talked no longer caring if he tore new, fragile skin. "Thank you for the referral. I hope this guy can help." The frustration and the discomfort he felt overwhelmed him as he wondered why specialists weren't called in from the beginning.

"Let me know how the appointment goes." Francine looked up as a patient in her office came up to the front desk.

"Okay, thanks again." Al made the call immediately, hoping as he dialed, that he remembered the correct number through all the discomfort he was suffering.

A friendly voice answered. "Dr. Groves's office."

Al breathed a sigh of relief and then spent close to an hour on the phone giving the office background on his condition. The initial appointment was scheduled far in advance due to Dr. Grove's desirability and reputation.

Al finished the call and decided to walk outside to get the

mail in the hope that the movement would take his mind off the itching. He didn't bother to grab a coat from the hook next to the back door. As he stepped onto the gravel driveway, he filled his lungs with the smell of the river behind their property.

The community where the house was located in Wayne had no sidewalk and consisted of country roads that would bend and twist to lend themselves to odd property shapes. Bob Evirdedis had coached Al to distinguish between gravel, grass, stone, and masonry as he maneuvered through the community and around his own property. The Lake Road home was a former lodge which utilized the river as a focal point and positioned the home's front to face the slow, moving water.

The two inches of snow that had fallen earlier that morning was still fresh. Distracted by the discomfort of his healing skin and forgetting the warning from Lee Peterson about the disorienting effects of accumulated snow, Al continued around the bend. He reached the mailbox precisely where he thought it should be and after reaching inside, dropped a couple of pieces in the snow. Bending down, his fingers started to get numb as he felt around in the snow until he was relatively sure he had retrieved all of that he thought might have dropped. Clutching the mail while he wrapped his arms around himself in the freezing weather, he turned to the right, to return the way he came around the driveway and neglected to count the steps. After several minutes, he realized that it was taking longer than it should have. Still taking into consideration the bend of the driveway and the fact that he thought he was almost to the kitchen stairs he walked solidly into a tree branch.

"Oww!" The needles of the white pine stabbed at his cheeks as the comforting smell of pine permeated his senses.

At least I'm still in Wayne.

Turning completely around, he walked forward, bent down to dig through the two inches of snow and felt asphalt. *Asphalt? I must be on the side of the road.*

Backing up, he bumped into another tree. He felt the trunk and realized it was the big oak across the street. Breathing deeply and shivering, he leaned against the tree and waited for rescue.

Elaine opened the kitchen door and began to scan the yard. She saw Al's shivering, coatless, figure across the street through the empty branches of forsythias at the edge of their property. "Al, what are you doing? It's freezing, come in!"

Al shook his head. "You stand there, keep yelling and eventually I'll make it home."

Elaine threw her coat on and then grabbed an additional one for Al. "I was going to leave you out here with your sarcasm." She threw the coat around his shoulders and put his left hand on her shoulder. "What were you thinking coming out here without your cane or coat?"

"Here." He pulled the mail out from the clutch of his right arm and handed it to her brusquely. "By the way, I dropped some. You might want to check." He let her lead him back toward the house. "I guess I had other things on my mind, but at least the itching eased a bit. I feel the cold all the way through me."

Elaine tucked the mail in her coat. "Let's get in the house."

The adventure reaffirmed the shock New Jersey's damp, cold, winters had on his injuries and recovery. The weather moved inside him as winter turned to spring that April. It took Mother Nature weeks to remove herself from deep within his body.

The scheduled appointment with Dr. Grove finally arrived April 11. Al and Elaine waited for over a half hour in the waiting room while Al squirmed in his chair. When the nurse called them, he rose quickly and Elaine had to toss the magazine she was reading on the weathered oak coffee table to keep up. Al let his cane and the sound of the nurse's voice guide him to an examination room at the end of the hall while Elaine followed two steps behind.

Once the nurse had shut the door, Al began to take off his oxford and T-shirt without prompting. She systematically asked all the necessary questions after checking his vital statistics as part of the exam preliminaries.

Dr. Grove walked into the room extending his hand first to Elaine and then reached down to take Al's. "I reviewed your case history sent over from Overlook Hospital and I am concerned that you are having all this discomfort while being treated." He looked at his patient seated on the examination table and took a brief inventory of the clothes lying next to him. "Where's your Jobe Shirt?"

Al contorted his face as he shifted on the table. "My what?"

"Your Jobe Shirt." Dr. Grove opened his eyes wide and looked at the two bewildered faces in front of him. "You two have no idea what I'm talking about?" He looked down at his chart. "That should have been sent home with you the day you left the hospital in November."

Al found his voice, but spoke with embarrassment barely above a whisper. "What is it?"

Dr. Grove shook his head slowly. "All of this discomfort could have been alleviated. A Jobe Shirt is a pressure garment that is elastic, one third the size of a normal shirt, and very tight. Putting it on is a struggle, but while you are wearing it, the shirt brings comfort from the constant itching and swelling of the scar tissue. This isn't magic, this is a pressure garment worn by all burn victims." Dr. Grove looked from Elaine to Al and then continued. "The success of a Jobe Shirt is from the pressure it applies to the injured area. The applied pressure replaces the permanently destroyed nerves at the injury location that had functioned as signals to the brain that the injured part of the body is finished healing and no longer needs the fluid and necessary nutrients. In some injury cases, the signal is only delayed or interrupted but in severe burns, such as in your case, some of the nerves are permanently destroyed. The pressure from the shirt that replaces these nerve signals works over the extended period of years.

Al straightened his back as he sat on the exam table. "Years?"

"Yes. I'm hoping that we can still minimize the permanent scarring in addition to giving you relief." Dr. Grove began to write on the chart he still held.

"If that thing is as small as you say, it would not have been

(171)

effective. It would have peeled off my healing skin." Al began to talk with his hands, something he had not done since before the accident.

Dr. Grove spoke as he continued to write. "The shirt is not pulled over your head, it is held in place with Velcro strips in the front. It does not peel healing skin. You should have been wearing this in the hospital. I read the records that were transferred to us." He moved over to the intercom system. "Carol? Please bring in a sample Jobe Shirt for Mr. Plevier." Dr. Grove caught the tall black stool on wheels with his foot and pulled it next to the examination table. "As you know from the experience of the trauma while healing from a burn, the skin reaches the point where it actually looks normal because the body has called for tissue to heal itself."

Al jumped into the doctor's monologue. "My wife said the skin looked almost translucent at one point."

Dr. Grove looked toward Elaine and reminded himself to take into consideration that the patient in front of him could not see his healing skin, he could only feel it. "The problem is that the body does not stop trying to heal the burn because the nerves that send the signal have been destroyed, allowing for an abundance of fluid and tissue which then creates scarring. The shirt will not stop all scarring but it will slow it down and minimize it." A nurse knocked, walked into the room and handed Dr. Grove what appeared to be a doll's shirt.

"Are you kidding me?" Elaine started to laugh as Dr. Grove held the shirt up to her and then handed it to Al to feel.

Al shook his head as he pulled at the doll size garment. "You have to be kidding me." He tossed it lightly to feel the weight and then became serious. "Why didn't someone tell us about this option before?"

The doctor looked at Elaine with a hard expression. "This is not an option. This is a necessity for any burn victim leaving the hospital. I'll attribute the doctor's lapse in judgment due to his primary objectives of keeping you alive and saving your eyes. I can't understand why this was not given to you during recent visits. It should have been the first avenue to pursue, especially with the discomfort you are in." He turned on the chair, opened a drawer and pulled out a prescription pad. "It's a shame that you have been suffering needlessly."

Al ran the fabric through his hands and then laid the shirt on his lap. "I'll never get into this thing."

"It only appears that way. Although it may feel thick to your finger as you touch it, when it is on your body it stretches so thin that it becomes like a second skin. You will have to struggle to get into it in the beginning, but after a few weeks of wearing one, you will be able to put it on without help from your wife." He smiled at Elaine for encouragement. "Now that you have felt it and have a basic introduction, let me conduct an examination." Dr. Grove rose from the stool.

Elaine was still bothered by the fact that in addition to all the pain that could have been avoided, he may have also suffered needlessly. "We did seek the advice of a dermatologist." Dr. Grove turned toward Elaine as she spoke. "He told Al the discomfort and pain he was feeling was in his mind due to the boredom of being stuck at home."

Dr. Grove shrugged his shoulders. "I guess I've heard it all."

Elaine sat straight in her chair, stoic and reserved. "Thank you for helping Al."

Al expressed his apprehension about the latest 'help' presented to them. "Will it be painful?"

"The exam, the fitting, or the shirt?" Dr. Grove, a patient man, was always professional.

"Any of them." Memories of debridement procedures and Mary flooded Al's brain.

"Please take off your pants and socks." Dr. Grove set the chart he had been continuously writing in on the counter and stood to begin his physical examination of Al. "No, the shirt will not hurt. You will feel almost instant relief when you put it on, to be accompanied by three days of intense itching and then on the third day, immediate and constant relief. The sensation of wearing a severely tight shirt is something you will look forward to, trust me.

(173)

The only time you will have the shirt off is to take a bath, and then it must be put back on immediately after patting your skin dry. Today I'm going to give you a prescription for mild soap to wash with. You cannot use any creams or lotions with the shirt. Are you currently using any prescribed creams or ointments now?"

Elaine spoke up from her chair. "No."

Dr. Grove turned to Elaine. "Will you be staying in the room during the exam?

Realizing she had spoken for Al, she turned to him. "Whatever you want, Al. Do you want to make sure I hear everything for the first visit?"

Al turned toward her. "Whatever the doctor feels will help. I'm fine either way."

A nurse entered and handed the Doctor more paperwork. "Thank you." After putting down the paperwork, Dr. Grove began to visually inspect Al as he spoke to Elaine. "You should stay. I may have questions from the original hospital stay that you can answer."

Al shifted on the examination table, unable to sit comfortably for long. "He's right, Elaine. I'm having a hard time concentrating."

"You will be sleeping better after you have a Jobe shirt. I see that the scarring on your legs is minimal." Dr. Grove lifted Al's arms to examine the worst area of destruction.

"My chest, arms, and back itch the worst. I hardly notice my legs." Al shifted as Dr. Grove touched his injuries.

"Have you had difficulty functioning with your hands?" He turned both Al's hands over and noticed no webbing. "I've never seen injuries of this magnitude without webbing on the hands.

Al nodded his head with pride. "The scars bothered me at home, initially, but I had such severe headaches and I was on such high doses of pain relievers, that I didn't pay much attention to it."

The doctor let go of his hands and Al clasped them defensively. "What about now?"

"The skin feels tight, but I assumed that was normal as part

(174)

the healing process considering how badly I was burned. I do anything I have the energy for and try to live with the pain. I can feel the dots on the Braille cards." Al smiled inside his head as he imagined the condition of the cards Lee Peterson had brought to him after Lee admitted he was one of the worst Braille students he ever had.

"Gloves are separate from the shirt, but my main concern is the scarring on the chest, under the right armpit and down the right arm." The doctor pressed on the scarred hands and asked Al how bad the pain was.

Al thought, "Not bad, really."

Dr. Grove lifted Al's arms. "The itching and swelling must be intolerable." He was still shocked that the man in front of him with such extensive burns was sent home without a Jobe Shirt. "Can you get into The City within the next day or two?" The doctor spoke over his shoulder to Elaine.

Elaine had become more confident in her driving since February, but still did not look forward to driving in Manhattan. "Yes, whatever it takes. Do we have to go to the hospital?"

"No. I need to send you for your first fitting to the company that makes the Jobe Shirt. We do not do that here. Nurses and trained medical staff who are very precise will fit you and will then order your shirts within two weeks. During the appointment where you receive the shirts, the nurses will give you instructions on the care of the shirts." Dr. Grove's exam moved to Al's torso. "You will need plastic surgery for the right side of your chest. Did Dr. Westmont talk to you about this?"

Elaine spoke up from behind the doctor. "No. Is there something that can be done?"

"The surgery is not elective. We have to rebuild the right side of his chest to eliminate the concave appearance and correct the damage caused by the chemical. This will take place next winter. I want you to use the Jobe Shirt and build up your strength first. Rebuilding the chest will be an invasive surgery. We have to take muscles and tissue from your back and shoulder and wrap them around." Dr. Grove gave Al a chance to absorb the what he

(175)

them, realizing it was an extensive amount of information. "Your file was very comprehensive in detail and enabled me to visualize most of the accident scene for myself."

Al was lost in his own thoughts as he tried to reconcile how doing the career he had chosen transformed into this lifetime of physical challenges and pain. "Do whatever you have to. I feel like I have no control over what happens to my body." Al spoke with resignation and surrender.

Dr. Grove looked from Al to Elaine and then continued with his part in Al's recovery. "I will want to see you in three weeks. Do you want me to prescribe something for the discomfort you are encountering until you get the shirt?"

"I'll use the drugs I already have." Al felt a cold instrument run on the top and underside of his feet.

"Do you feel what I am doing?" The doctor continued to prod Al's feet.

Al reflexively jerked his foot slightly. "You're running something cold on my feet."

"Does the instrument feel cold on the top and bottom of your foot?" Dr. Grove looked at the minuscule amount of webbing between the toes and expected more damage.

"I feel it on the top and bottom. I only had trouble walking right after I came home." Al felt the doctor stop. "The headaches were so severe that I ignored my feet."

"Aside from the webbing and the expected scarring, I have to say you are extremely lucky." Dr. Grove stepped away from Al and looked at the spots of scar tissue on his right leg.

Al didn't know whether to laugh or cry. "I'm glad to be alive, but I would have felt luckier if I had my sight."

The doctor closed his eyes to reflect as he stood before his patient and the wife who had endured so much. "I understand. All things considered, you must have an angel looking out for you." Dr. Grove looked over at the Jobe Shirt still sitting on the examination table next to Al. "How do you feel about the material of the Jobe Shirt? It's lightweight and won't be anything other than restrictive on your skin."

Al paused before responding. "I'll have to take your word. I wish my angel had given me more warning that day. My free will might have decided differently." He tried not to sound jaded.

The doctor looked toward Elaine apologetically, afraid he may have made his patient feel worse instead of giving him hope. "You're alive and to be quite frank, drawing my own conclusions from your records, you shouldn't be. You have a strong will to live. I read that you had facial burns, but I only see scarring on your forehead and scalp."

Elaine joined the conversation and hoped to divert the anger she could see rising in Al. "The first time I saw him in the hospital, he looked like a black pumpkin. He did not have lips. I remember thinking that it was bad enough he couldn't see, but did he have to look like a monster too?"

"Thanks, Dear." Al smiled and laughed, immediately breaking the tension in the room.

Elaine looked over at Al's smile. "The swelling started to go down within the first week, and by the time we brought him home his face was still puffy and red, but the skin was no longer black."

"Did you have plastic surgery done to the facial area while at Overlook?"

Al answered. "No, but now that we've met, I'll give you a call after the crow's feet start." He began to feel his sense of humor return. Al reached for his t-shirt where he had placed it next to him.

The doctor watched Al put it on. "You should always have a shirt on. This is not just while you're healing, but anytime. Spend as little time as possible in direct sunlight, always staying under some type of cover."

Al shifted on the table. "I have no desire to go to the beach, but the cold bothers me. Will it always be this way?"

"The cold may continue to bother you, and you will probably enjoy the warmer weather." He looked from Elaine to Al. "Any other questions?"

"Do you have any idea why my hair is so much oilier?" Al

touched his head for effect. "Elaine tells me the color has changed too. I used to be a towhead."

"It could be a number of factors, but the simplest reason I could give you is that your body had been through a tremendous battle for survival and is reacting in its own way." He inclined his head toward the medical chart he had been writing in. "I see the pain medications you mentioned are listed in your records. Is that for the headaches or for the discomfort from the burns?"

Al became defensive. "I only use the pain medication if my headaches become unbearable. The doctor prescribed Valium to calm me for the itching and pain, but I would prefer not to be on them any longer."

"Good. I don't mind if you use something at night, after all, you do need to rest, but the medication should be a bridge and not a crutch. The Jobe Shirt is what you need for constant relief and long-term healing." The doctor sat on the black stool and placed both hands on his knees like a catcher waiting for the next throw.

Elaine caught the comical display and drew everyone's attention back to the Jobe Shirt. "Dr. Grove, is the shirt covered by insurance?"

"It should be. Check with my receptionist to be certain. This is an integral part of Albert's recovery and the insurance companies I've dealt with in the past have always covered the expense 100 percent. I'll write a prescription for two and the company in Manhattan can submit it to your carrier. You'll need two shirts so that after you hand wash one and hang it to dry, you'll still have the other. Remember, you are never to be without it, even when you sleep. Never put the shirts on wet or damp." He looked over at Elaine. "The fabric is very lightweight and despite the strength of the elastic, it allows air to pass through to your skin." He gathered his paperwork and prepared to end the visit as he reached into a drawer and handed a brochure to Elaine. "This is the Jobe Shirt manufacturing company, their address, and phone number. I will have the receptionist call them and schedule their first available appointment." Dr. Grove carefully accepted the Al's extended right hand.

"Take care folks. I will see you in three weeks." He closed the door quietly as he left.

Elaine walked over and grabbed the Jobe Shirt from Al. "This feels like a girdle."

Al smiled. "How would you know what a girdle feels like with your figure?"

"It feels like another layer of skin. How is this thing ever going to fit over your torso? It looks like a doll's shirt." Elaine pulled at the garment.

"I don't know. To be honest, it scares me. After I have it on for the week, I can tell Dr. Grove what I think of it." Al reached to his left and retrieved his coat with a smirk on his face. "I think that went well. Now I get to feel like a sausage, and it will still itch and hurt."

"Only the second and third day. Be patient and stop with the analogies. You're annoying." Elaine helped Al with his jacket.

"Aren't you a sweetheart." Al buttoned his jacket. "Summer should be pleasant. I'll have another layer of skin."

She rolled her eyes and laughed harder. "He said the shirt breathes." Elaine retrieved her coat and handed Al his cane.

"Nothing keeps a good man down." He smiled and held the door open for Elaine.

Walking down the short corridor to the waiting room, the receptionist greeted them. "I set up the appointment with the Jobe Shirt manufacturer for tomorrow at eleven o'clock. Does that work for you?"

"That will be fine, thank you." Elaine cringed inwardly at the thought of the drive into Manhattan, but at least the appointment time was after the morning commuter traffic. She took two appointment cards from the young woman, one for the Jobe Shirt and one for the next appointment with Dr. Grove in three weeks. "Do we need to bring anything with us to the Jobe Shirt fitting?"

"No. Do you have the address and directions?" The receptionist looked only at Elaine.

(179)

"I have the brochure, thank you." Elaine and Al left the office two hours after their arrival.

The ride home was intolerable, as Al remained in the back seat alternating between sitting and lying down. He walked the yard in circles trying to take his mind off his healing skin. He practiced in the cool air that attacked his skin until he heard the phone ring through the open kitchen window.

Elaine found Al counting his steps between the garage, the kitchen, and the mailbox. "You have that area memorized. What are you doing?" She watched how uncomfortable he was and wondered how he would survive until he had the Jobe shirt.

"Trying to occupy my mind. I'm going to walk the perimeter of the property next. I'd jump into the river if I thought I could swim alone." Al kept walking as he spoke. "Who was on the phone?"

"A buyer for the Tempest. He saw the ad in last week's paper and wanted to know if late this afternoon worked to look at it. I told them to come over in an hour." Elaine hugged herself against the late afternoon chill.

"That's fine. Is eighty dollars good? That's all I think its worth." Al felt the cold, but wasn't ready to go inside.

"Whatever you think." Elaine hugged herself tighter and turned to walk back into the house. "I'm going to get my coat. Are you sure you want to be alone with the buyer if I go pick up Albert?"

Al called loudly after her. "I'll take care of this. You've dealt with enough and I don't want to come in yet. The title's in the kitchen drawer next to the sink. Can you get it for me?" Al waited and paced, running his hand along the station wagon as he walked and heard Elaine closing the kitchen window.

She came out and handed the car title to Al. "Here you go. You sure you don't want me to be here with you?" She was secretly glad not to have to deal with the car herself but didn't want Al to think she was dumping it on him.

"Nah, I got it." He stepped along the driveway and then started toward the two-car detached garage.

She watched his body twitch as he walked. "I'll be back in an hour with Albert. I think mom fed him already. Maybe you and I can have pizza." Elaine reached around him for the door handle.

"Whatever you think. My mind is not on food. All I can think about is that shirt." He kissed her lightly and then stepped back to let her drive away.

Al counted his steps to the garage, found his way to the passenger side of the Pontiac Tempest and leaned his cane near the front tire. He cleaned out the glove box while he waited and a short time later heard a car pull onto the gravel driveway. Climbing out of the Tempest, he walked to the front of the car and sat on the hood. Two car doors opened, he heard two sets of feet cross the front yard, and approach the Tempest.

"Are you Mr. Plevier?" A man's voice spoke to him.

"That's me." Al extended his right hand not realizing he extended it away from the man who was speaking.

The man reached over and took his hand. "Is this the car?"

"This is it," Al responded and stepped away from the hood. "Do you want to take her for a ride?"

"Maybe. This is a good-looking car. How does it run?" Al heard the man walk around the driver's side door and open it.

"It runs good. I'm asking eighty dollars for it." Al started to walk to the driver's side door running his hand along the hood for guidance.

"Would you take sixty for it? I need a second car for my wife and the kids." The buyer shut the car door.

Al took a deep breath and decided it was ridiculous to argue over twenty dollars. "My wife's not home, but I guess she wouldn't mind. It was her car originally and now since my accident, we only need the wagon for our family. I want it out of the garage." Al pulled the title out of his pocket, already signed. "Sixty dollars, please."

Al held out his hand as the man counted out the money and placed it in his palm. "Twenty, forty, and sixty dollars."

Al smiled good-naturedly at the man. "Nice doing business

(181)

with you. Thanks." He then walked around the front and retrieved his cane.

The buyer had taken the title from Al, quickly threw license plates he had brought with him on the dash and rear window, and once Al had moved away started the engine.

"You got plates with you?" Al asked as he heard the engine starting knowing Elaine had already removed and returned the plates to the New Jersey Division of Motor Vehicles.

"We threw them on already." The other car started and without saying goodbye, both cars pulled away quickly.

Al was left standing in the driveway. *That was weird and fast. The person with him never said a word. Whatever…I got my money and I never really liked that car anyway. I should have gotten rid of it a long time ago.* Al counted his steps back to the kitchen door when he felt the itching begin with ferocity and inadvertently his cane hit the bottom step with a loud thwack. *And that's why you never leave the house without your cane. That could have been my face.*

He went into the kitchen to wait for Elaine. A short time later, she walked in with the baby. "Hi, Al. I see the Tempest is gone." Albert ran past his dad for the toy pile in his bedroom.

Al held out the cash. "Here you go, Sweetie. Don't spend it all in one place."

Elaine looked at the money Al had handed her. "Al, how much did you sell the car for?"

Al was surprised she cared about twenty dollars. "Sixty dollars. I didn't feel like arguing with the guy over twenty dollars if it meant that much to him."

"Al," Elaine paused. "There's only thirty dollars here."

He couldn't believe it and jumped up off the chair. "What! I should have given him the car. I hope he needed that thirty dollars bad enough to screw over a blind guy!" Much to his own surprise, Al was not embarrassed, but instead, he was red hot mad.

Elaine was careful. "I'm glad you got that thing out of my garage. I almost had it towed."

"I know, but these dirtbags have to be kidding!" Al was

(182)

getting angrier as he stood before his wife and then remembered he didn't even bother to get the buyer's name.

Elaine worked to diffuse Al's anger, but not at the expense of his pride. "I'm sure you'll invent ways to circumvent situations that leave you vulnerable to the world." Al was silent as she turned to make dinner for her family. "I haven't heard you complain about your burns for five minutes. Maybe I should hunt the guy down and thank him." Elaine looked anxiously at Al.

"I think it was the feeling of cash in my hand. It really does have the power to heal." Al ran his hand over his chest as he calmed himself down. "That will never happen again." He scratched lightly at his chest after the affirmation spoken with deadly calm and then finished with usual humor. "Things could have been worse. It could have been three ones."

Chapter XV: Faith and Grace

Elaine and Al arrived at the Jobe Shirt manufacturer in Manhattan, the lesson of yesterday filed away in both of their memories for future use. They were called into the patient fitting room immediately as three technicians followed behind them.

One technician was the obvious lead for the procedure and did not waste any time. "In order to measure you for the fitting, you need to take off your shirt. Your pants and shoes can remain on, but you will need to unbutton the waistband. The Jobe Shirt will come down to the top of your hip bone." The lead technician began to unfold the material she had draped over her arm.

"Do you need me to sit on an examination table?" He felt as if he was about to be on display.

The same technician spoke to him as she moved to his right. "No. You need to be in a standing position in order to take the measurements."

He heard several voices talking around him to each other. "Who is in the room?"

The head technician, in her haste, hadn't taken into consideration that the patient before her could not see. "I'm sorry,

(184)

Mr. Plevier. We will explain the steps in more detail for you so it is clear. Three of us will be needed for the measuring. I am Bea, and I have my two assistants, Emily and Sharon."

Al relaxed a little as he began to unbutton his shirt. "Thank you. I understand that you ladies have a lot of work ahead of you, but I would appreciate it if you could explain what you are doing as we go along." The coolness of the room attacked his scarred skin and he felt himself shiver.

Bea held strips of paper in front of Elaine, who had tried to find a corner of the room to stand in. "Mrs. Plevier, this is the paper we use with the rubber bands to get the proper measurement." She turned back to Al and saw him react to the temperature in the room. "We will try to get you through this as quickly as possible, Mr. Plevier. Would you like to hold one of the strips of paper so that you can get the idea of what we are trying to achieve?" She placed the paper into his hands without waiting for a reply.

He felt the paper and rubbed it between his fingers. "It feels like it could tear easily."

The technicians finished laying out the paper strips and bands and prepared to start. "It's strong enough don't worry. We're going to get started now. If you feel strange, cold or uncomfortable in any manner, please tell us and we can stop and explain what we're doing."

Al hugged his injured torso. "I'm cold right now."

The three technicians worked steadily measuring the strips of paper. "We're sorry and we'll get through this as quickly as possible, but it has to be done right the first time. If the shirt is not fitted properly, it can't do its job."

Al uncrossed his arms and dealt with the chilly air. "Understood."

"Mrs. Plevier, if you have any questions please feel free to ask. I understand that this is new to you." Bea directed her next comment to Al. "It's a shame you weren't given the Jobe Shirt initially, but at least you're here now. You'll notice an immediate positive change in your recovery." She stood back to examine the progress so far.

Emily spoke as she looked Al over carefully. "Albert, lift both arms out to your sides and stand like the letter T."

Al raised his arms as high as his injuries would allow and felt strips of paper go down the length of each arm. Smaller strips of the same type paper were then wrapped around each arm and overlapped each other from the shoulder to the wrist. Each strip was fastened into place with tape and rubber bands. He began to drop his arms and Sharon saw his confusion and calmly stopped him. "Please keep your arms extended a few more minutes."

The technicians wrapped larger pieces of paper around his torso and back. These sections were fastened into place with tape. After the measurements were finished, a template was created for the shirt. The entire procedure took a half hour and then ended anticlimactically with Al given permission to dress.

Bea gave the final nod of conclusion. "You can relax now. We have all the measurements we need." She wrote notes while the two assistants bagged all the utilized material. "The shirt should be ready in a week. Before you leave, schedule an appointment to come back for the fitting."

Elaine spoke from behind the women. "Can it be mailed to us?" She realized from the expression on all of their faces that her question was naïve.

"No." Bea was patience but firm. "We will have to teach you how to put it on. It's a challenge, but not impossible and you will need our instructions the first time."

Al reached for his shirt still on the examination table, eager to get out of the cold, antiseptic fitting room. "We're finished for today?"

Bea smiled, "That's it. You two have a safe drive home." All three women smiled and left the room.

He turned in Elaine's direction knowing she would need some time to relax after the drive into the city. "Do you want to get some lunch before you have to drive home? It might be nice to sit at a neighborhood café."

She stood up and carried Al's cane to him. "I'd rather just

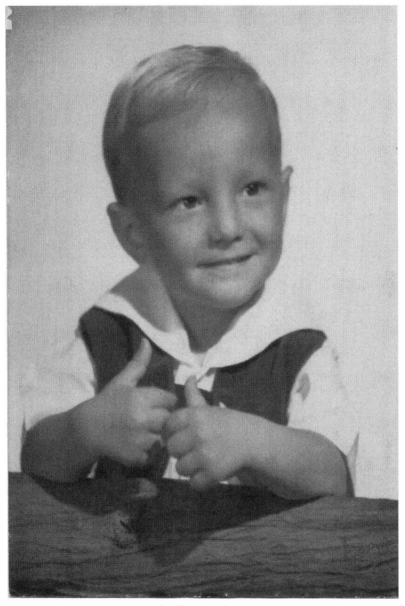

*Al age two, 1952. Thumbs up and
ready to take on the world.*

(187)

Jayne Kelly

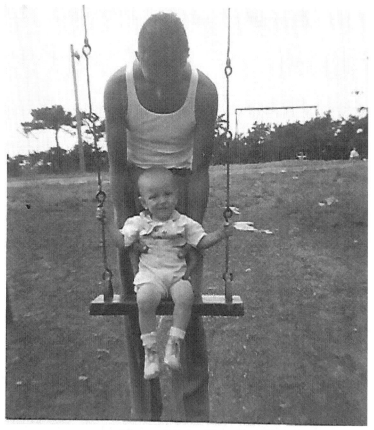

Al and his Dad. 1951

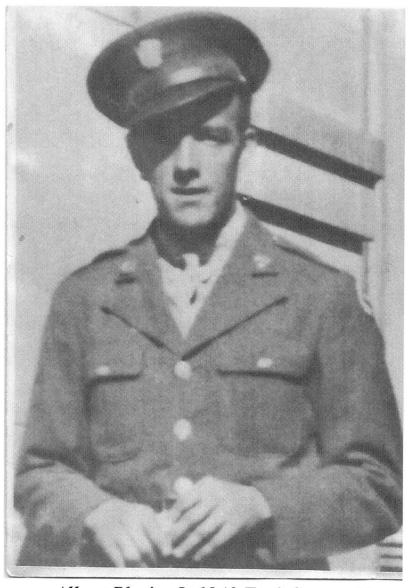

Albert Plevier I: 1943 Tech Sgt.   Mortar Division US Army

Jayne Kelly

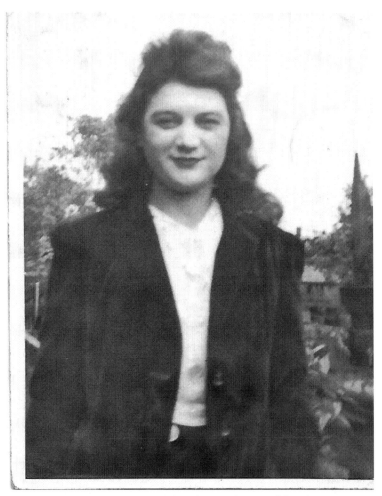

Rose Plevier circa 1940

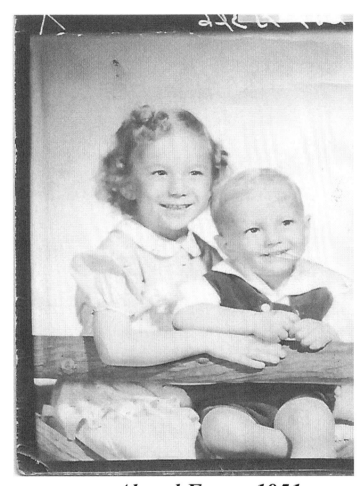

Al and Fenna 1951

Jayne Kelly

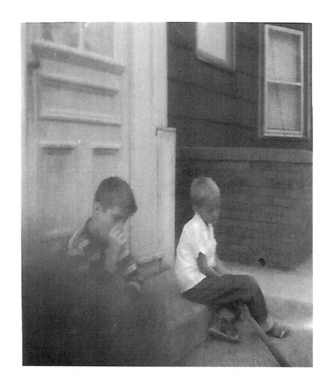

Paterson Stickball Dugout

(192)

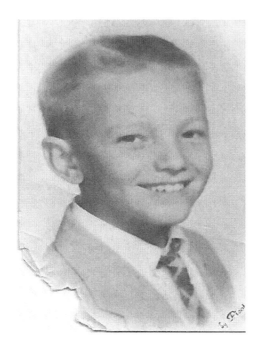

1960

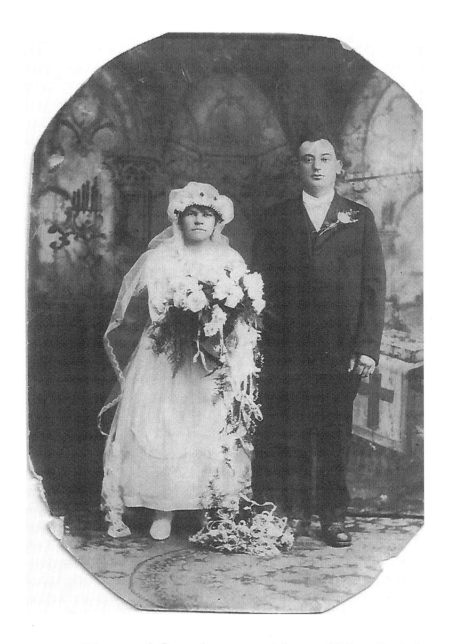

Maternal Grandparents: Mr. and Mrs. Padula

(194)

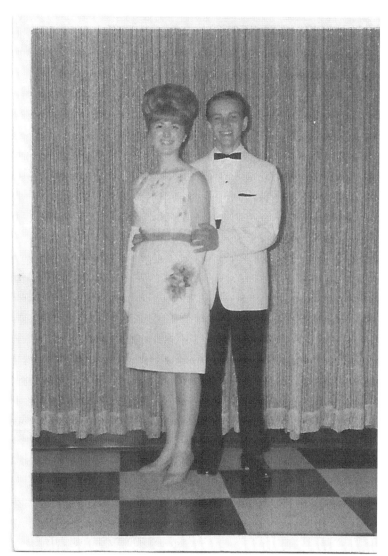

High School Prom

(195)

Jayne Kelly

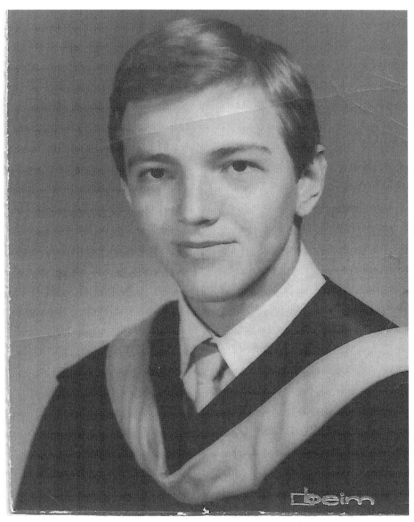

Newark College of Engineering
Graduation 1971

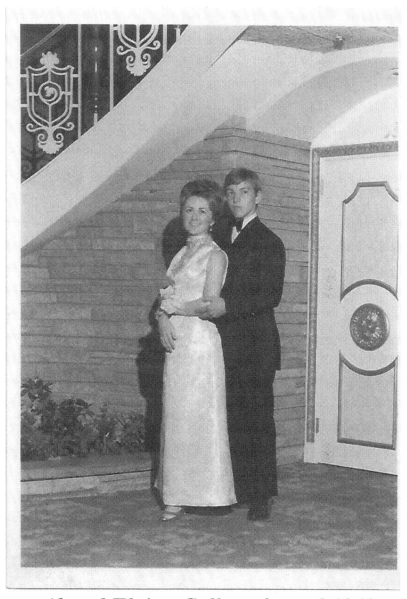

Al and Elaine College formal 1969

(197)

Jayne Kelly

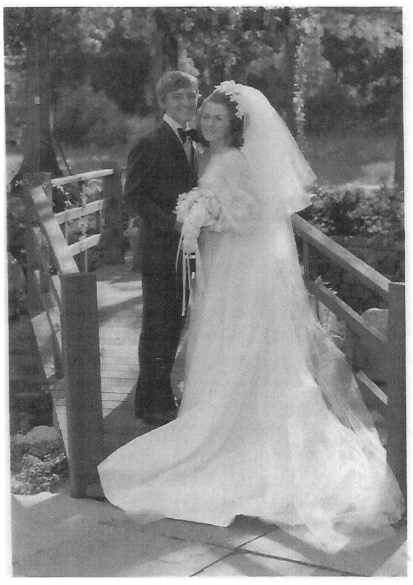

Mr. and Mrs. Albert Plevier   June 19, 1971

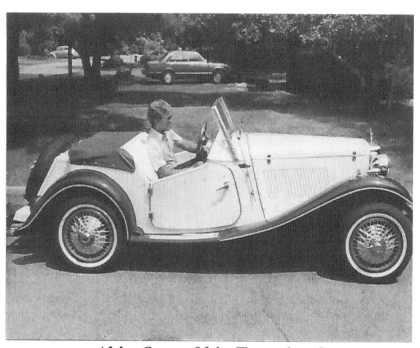

Al in One of his Favorite Cars

get it over with and hit the road."

Al held out his hand to her. "Let's go."

He spent the following week feeling as though his itching was even more exaggerated than before. Part of him attributed this to the anticipation of the immediate relief only days away. He maintained a countdown by marking off each passing day in his own mind until the call came that the shirts were ready.

During the drive into Manhattan to pick up the shirts, Al squirmed continuously. "This is unbearable. Today has been the worst."

Elaine tried to concentrate on maneuvering through the Lincoln Tunnel. "You'll get the relief you need shortly." *Me too.* She thought privately.

Al stopped moving abruptly. "I hope you're right."

Elaine looked over at his aggravated posture. "It will work."

She found parking, relieved the trip had ended. "We're going to have to walk three blocks."

Al almost jumped out of the car. "That's not too bad for Manhattan. How do you feel after this latest drive in The City?" The generic term for Manhattan borough by natives of New Jersey interchanged easily for them.

Elaine breathed out. "I'm always glad when it's over." She met Al at the front of the car and looked at his empty hands. "Where's your cane?"

He shook himself, realizing how distracted the discomfort had made him. "I'll get it."

"The car's locked. Stay where you are." Al was too uncomfortable to make conversation, and Elaine was already thinking about the return trip home.

"I hope this appointment goes as quickly as the last one." He tried to sound nonchalant as his desire to begin this part of his recovery grew.

The receptionist looked up from her paperwork and stood to greet them in the empty waiting room. "Hi, Mr. and Mrs. Plevier. You can come into the examination room. Please take off your shirt and t-shirt." The receptionist left and the same technicians from last week entered.

Bea spoke first. "Good Morning." She carried two tiny shirts.

Elaine put a hand in front of her mouth to suppress a laugh. "Oh Al, the shirts look like they're made for dolls."

Al unbuttoned his Oxford shirt, slipped it off with his T-shirt, and prepared for the worst. "This should be pleasant." One technician carrying a Jobe Shirt approached Al and placed it in his hands and handed the second shirt to Elaine.

Al burst out laughing. "You have to be kidding me. These feel smaller than the one Dr. Grove handed me at his office."

Bea kept her professional demeanor. "It will work and the relief you'll feel will be nothing short of amazing. We'll do this one arm at a time, and we'll start with your left." Bea took the shirt from Al and began to ball up the left sleeve.

Al stopped the procedure to gently remind the technicians he couldn't see them. "Is that you Bea?"

Bea realized she had forgotten the courtesy of introduction to her new patient who didn't have sight. "Yes, Mr. Plevier, I apologize. Emily and Sharon are here also." She had the shirt sleeve balled up she placed it over his hand and began to work it upward. "Relax your hand and don't clench it into a fist."

Al felt like he was being worked over in a prize fight. "You guys don't waste any time. I thought you'd give me a minute to gather some courage." He relaxed his hand as the restrictive material was unrolled upward. The material closed tightly over his wrist leaving him to wonder how he would survive with it wrapped around his body. "Will I be able to breathe normally? You're never going to get that over my whole arm, never mind the rest of me."

"We will work one inch at a time. You're not our first patient." The technicians attempt to relax him had little effect. "Mrs. Plevier you should help today. This will be a two, person job until Al can manage it alone. It could take him weeks of practice before he can put the Jobe Shirt on unaided." Bea was at

(201)

the elbow after a rough jerking movement upward that brought Al onto his toes.

He grunted accordingly. "I'm going to lose the feeling in my arm. You're putting me in a vise grip." He began to unintentionally squirm away from the women.

"Try to stand still. Once you start to feel relief from the burns, you'll look forward to wearing this." She returned to jerking, pulling and rolling the sleeve over his arm.

"Easy, Bea." *I'm ripping' this off the minute I get home.* With memories of Mary never far away while he was undergoing any medical procedure, Al was afraid the women would retaliate if he voiced his thoughts.

Bea could see the discomfort and frustration on Al's face and knew from past experience what this patient was thinking. "Leave the shirt at night. It has to start doing its job. The only time it should be off is when you bathe." Bea had reached Al's left shoulder and began to pull and stretch the material to reach his right arm. "Elaine, come over here and pull as hard as you can, holding the shirt over his shoulder as I roll the sleeve over his right arm beginning at the hand."

Elaine pulled as directed and began to feel sorry for Al. "Oh, my God, we're going to dislocate his shoulder."

Bea maintained control of the fitting. "Al, relax your left arm and shoulder and let them hang loosely at your side."

"This thing is cutting off my circulation." Al clenched and unclenched his fists in an attempt to keep blood flowing.

Together Bea and Elaine reached his right hand, balled up the sleeve and began to facilitate its ascent. "If you can squeeze your shoulder blades together, it would help. I understand the severity of your injuries, but this will not cause further damage. Elaine, you and I are going to switch places so that you can learn how to bring the sleeve over the arm." One of the technicians came over to aid in the transfer and assist as the shirt continued to pull Al's shoulder blades together. Bea released the sleeve to Elaine who almost lost it as the elasticity snapped. "You're doing great."

Al grunted while he tried to maintain his balance as Bea and Emily pulled at the shirt and Elaine worked the sleeve. "Can she practice on a dummy first?"

"I already am." Sweat began to gather on her forehead as she worked the material up to his elbow at a much slower pace than that of the technician.

Bea watched Elaine work the material over Al's arm until finally, Emily could release her hold. "Good. How does that feel, Mr. Plevier?"

"Like my arms are in girdles. You have to be a contortionist to pull this off." Al tried to relax his shoulders back to their normal position, but found that what should have been a simple movement was now a task. "My back is fighting the shirt already."

I'm definitely not bothering with this thing after I get home.

"The Velcro straps that fasten in the front are wide so that they will be strong enough to withstand the elasticity and pull of the shirt. Elaine, you will help with the front now." Bea stepped aside to allow room. The two women pulled and fastened the Velcro from the bottom upward until the shirt was secured.

Sharon, the third technician, spoke for the first time as the four women looked Al over. "Bea, we have a perfect fit."

Bea stood back. "Yes, perfect!"

Al struggled to get used to the constricting shirt on his chest. "I can hardly move in this not to mention breathe." He stiffly moved his arms for effect.

"You'll get used to it. While wearing the shirt, you will want to continue with your daily routines. Taking it off and on is not an option." Bea began to walk around Al and examine all sides with her two colleagues.

Elaine watched the look on Al's face. "Does he have to go through this every day?"

"Yes. If you want the desired results, there is no compromise." Bea inclined her head. "You will get used to it. It will be like having a second skin and believe it or not you will look forward to putting it back on after you bathe."

Al stopped trying to move his arms. "I don't know if any of you will believe me, but I feel better right now." Relief spread over his face.

Sharon looked toward Elaine and smiled. "We expected that. Normally you will feel instant relief that lasts throughout the first day." Sharon paused for effect before continuing. "However, the second and third days are torturous. After you get through them, you will feel as good as you do right now."

Elaine stared at Al in disbelief. "Dr. Grove mentioned this to us, but would you mind explaining it further? Why would he have more discomfort for two days than he has had for the last year and then return to bliss?"

Bea pulled down on the bottom to the shirt to adjust a ripple and spoke directly toward Al. "You have a lot of fluid that has built up and must be reabsorbed into the body. After the majority of fluid has been redistributed you will have relief. The applied constant pressure sends a signal to the brain that the area is healed. This overrides the destroyed nerves that can no longer send signals. My suggestion for the next forty-eight hours is to rely on the pain medication you were previously given and to remember that the unpleasant discomfort is temporary."

Al ran his hands over the shirt. "I may actually sleep on the car ride home."

Bea spoke directly to Al. "Be prepared for tomorrow."

"Let me enjoy today, please. I'll worry about tomorrow, tomorrow." Al reached for his white undershirt but struggled with the new arm constrictions.

Elaine automatically reached out to help get the T-shirt over his arms. "I'm sure you'll be doing this yourself tomorrow."

"Thanks, Sweetheart." Al pulled the undershirt down his body and then struggled on his own to slip into the oxford shirt.

Elaine saw a new freedom as she watched Al move his body without discomfort. "Let's get out of here. How about lunch in the city? Last time we skipped it."

"Sounds good." He felt his cane placed in his right hand.

Elaine looked toward Bea. "Do you forward the bill to the

insurance company or do I take care of that?"

"We bill the insurance and let you know if a problem occurs with the carrier. You'll have copies of all the invoices mailed to your home."

Bea finished the last statement and saw Al grasp Elaine's hand. "You're not quite ready to go. We should now go over care of the shirt and what you will need to do for the next three days. We'll get you out of here as quickly as possible." She confirmed that she had their undivided attention and watched Al. "You cannot take the Jobe shirt off for the next three days. That means no bathing."

He placed his cane next to him and started to fasten the buttons on his shirt that he had neglected. "No showering for three days? I'll be nice and ripe." *I can put up with anything as long as I have this relief.*

"I know you were told not to wear deodorant today, but you cannot use any deodorant for the duration that you wear the shirts. The products can harm the shirts integrity." Bea stared directly into Elaine's eyes.

Now Al began to worry about the tradeoff of comfort for hygiene. "What? How can I walk around in public without deodorant for two to three years?"

"Baby powder is absorbent and will not harm the suit. You will be surprised how well it works. The only time the shirt should be off after the next three days is when you are bathing. Then, dry yourself off by patting your torso with a towel and put the shirt right back on. No creams or lotions of any kind. You will have two shirts. If one is being washed, you will have a second to put on. The shirt should be washed with only a mild soap like the type you use for your toddler. Rinse the shirt and then lay it flat to dry. The shirts are very thin and consequently dry quickly. Do not wear one if it is partially damp. Make sure the shirt is completely dry. Stay out of the sun and if you are outside, try to stay under some cover. Above all, you have to remember to keep it on constantly. Your body needs the constant pressure and time. This is a long process. The next two days will be the hardest, but then it will be

(205)

a routine without the discomfort. We want to hear from you in three weeks to follow your progression. When is your appointment with the plastic surgeon?' Bea directed her questions to Elaine.

"In two weeks." Elaine's stomach growled and she gratefully looked forward to eating in Manhattan and not rushing back to Wayne.

"That's fine. Please make sure to call us with any questions. It was a pleasure to work with both of you." Bea extended her hand first to Elaine and then grasped Al's.

"Good luck to you, Mr. Plevier." The other two women almost spoke at the same time before offering their hands too.

If one more person wishes me good luck, I'm going to wonder if that's all I'm living off of.

The door shut quietly. "Why didn't we follow them out?"

"I'm writing in the notebook about the visit and the Jobe shirt details. Give me a minute." She wrote her last note and closed the book.

"You're precise with that, aren't you?" Pride mixed with annoyance as Al waited to escape the confines of the building and enjoy the new freedom the shirt gave him. He grabbed his cane and took a step toward the door.

"We can't forget anything. The smallest detail could be significant at some later date." She closed the book and tucked it into her purse.

After a leisurely two-hour lunch in the city, the car ride to Wayne was almost carefree with Al sitting in the front next to Elaine and talking nonstop. He made jokes that refreshed the banter between them, causing smiles on both their faces. For the first time since the accident, the family enjoyed an evening at home without medical drama and Al fully present. He fell into bed that night still wearing the Jobe Shirt and drifting into a deep, comfortable sleep, unaided by medication. He hardly noticed the constrictive material on his torso and arms.

Morning came too soon. The accompanying itching and pain the plastic surgeon and technicians had warned him about woke him out of a deep sleep with a vengeance. He stumbled out of bed and found his way to a wall as Elaine looked on from the doorway.

"I'm back where I started, except this is worse. I can't stand it." Al stood in the door frame in the master bedroom and rubbed his back up and down on top of the Jobe shirt. "The nurses were right. The pain and itching are worse than before. I don't know how much of it I can take."

"You want codeine?" Elaine watched him with mixed feelings.

"Yes. Give me as many as I'm allowed. I wish I could go back to sleep and wake up in three days." He heard Elaine's feet pad across the carpet away from him. He continued to rub against the door frame until he heard her coming back.

"Here." She placed two pills in his left hand and a paper cup with water in the other. "Al, don't take them dry, the pills might get stuck in your throat."

He quickly threw down the pills with the water and then walked to the bed, falling onto his back and rolling around like a dog with fleas. "I'm going to be a mess when this is over. Strung out from pills, lack of sleep, and smelling like roadkill."

"We'll get through this." Elaine stopped.

In six hours, he awoke and rubbed against any piece of wall or furniture he could find. "I feel like an injured bear."

"Don't hurt your new skin. Do you want something to eat?" Elaine didn't know what to do for him.

"No, I don't think I can keep anything down. As soon as I can have more pills, let me." Al walked away from the kitchen and then turned back. "Maybe, if I go outside the air will help. Where's my cane?"

"You left it next to the back door yesterday." Elaine looked at her husband in the sweatpants and shirt from yesterday.

Al found the cane exactly where he had left it. "I'm going to walk around the driveway a couple of hundred times, not down the street. The neighbors will call the cops if someone finds me rubbing my back against a tree or the other side of their house."

"We should call the doctor." She watched Al walk out the

door as she placed Albert into his high chair.

Fifteen minutes later Al was walking in the back door. "I'm coming out of my skin. Give me more pills."

"You should eat something first. I know you're not hungry, but you can't take this stuff on an empty stomach. Watch the baby while I get the medication. Albert is still in his high chair." Elaine brought back the pills and found Al rubbing against the wall and Albert giggling nonstop. "How about a peanut butter and jelly sandwich?"

"Fine, whatever. I don't care." Al ate the sandwich and then washed down pills with juice. He walked as far as the couch in the living room, lay down, writhed against the cushions and then passed out.

For the next two days and nights, Al and Elaine slept apart for the second time in their marriage. It was a difficult three days for the entire family due to a combination of his extreme discomfort, lack of bathing and unpleasant mood. On the third day, Al felt sick from the medication and decided he would wait for the miracle hour to come around when the shirt's abilities came to fruition. While waiting, he did not sit down for more than five minutes. Pacing the driveway began to make him dizzy, so he walked the property line over and over in only his Jobe shirt and pants. The weather had been unseasonably warm with bright sunshine, and against doctor's orders, he went outside without cover. The sun beat down on his shoulders and the irritation countered the itching and pain, leaving him to choose the lesser of two evils.

Just for today, just for today. The sun in small increments. I know it could hurt me, but just for today. It feels good on my face. How many more hours of this can I stand? I'll never sleep tonight unless I take those pills.

Elaine yelled from the back door. "Al, Dr. Grove is on the phone. Do you want to talk to him?" Elaine knew the answer.

"You talk to him." Al continued his walk around their yard and heard Elaine finally close the door.

He came into the house three hours later and went to bed,

falling into a disruptive yet exhaustive sleep. At seven o'clock the next morning, Elaine awakened to the sound of the shower running. She went into the master bath and found the beige Jobe shirt on the floor and her husband in the shower. "Al?"

He finished rinsing his head, grabbing to the right for a clean towel from the shelf. "The itching stopped, but I need you to help me get into the other shirt. This one smells."

Elaine stood in shock. "I'll get it."

Al felt for the clean boxers he had left on the sink and slipped them on. "I think you'll have to burn the clothes I've been wearing. This was a rough couple of days for all of us." He patted himself down with a generous amount of baby powder while waiting.

Elaine walked into the bathroom and stood in front of her husband. "Here's the other shirt. How do you want to start this?"

"We'll do it the same as we did in the office. I want to get that thing back on as quickly as possible. It feels good." Al reached in front of himself, toward his wife and the shirt.

"Here. Put your right hand out. I'll bunch the sleeve and roll it up your arm." Elaine started working the garment over Al's hand.

"Rolling it won't work. We'll have to keep stretching it. You have it over the wrist, keep going." Al tried to push into the sleeve to help her.

"Good. You push and I'll pull." Elaine stepped behind Al's right shoulder to get a better grip. "This is taking too long. We've got to get this thing on." Al grabbed hold of the right side of the shirt and tried to stretch the material.

Elaine jumped in. "Not yet. Wait until we have the right arm all the way in." She got the sleeve to the shoulder. "Now bring your arm back, after I bunch the left sleeve."

After getting the left arm in, Al tried to pull the shirt closed by bending over and squeezing his arms together. Elaine laughed with abandon at the sight of him, until he couldn't help but join her.

"I'm a contortionist. Maybe you can sell me to the circus."

(209)

Together Al and Elaine pulled the shirt closed and fastened the Velcro.

Elaine stepped back to take a look. "I'm sweating. That's a workout for me too. How do you feel now that you're wearing the shirt?"

"I feel the same way I did the day I left the office in The City." Al moved his arms around for effect. "It works. Now that I smell pretty, how about a kiss to rejuvenate me?"

Elaine gave him a kiss and ran her hands over the shirt. "This is like another layer of skin."

"You're right." Al moved his body around in the shirt. "I feel like I can finally think clearly."

They heard Little Albert called to his mother. "I need to see what he's up to." She wrapped her arms around the shirt and squeezed her husband lightly before leaving.

Al tried to lift his arms. "Don't forget me in here. I may need to be rescued."

Elaine walked into the nursery and smiled at Albert. "Good morning cutie." She raised the blinds and let in the streaming sunshine.

Chapter XVI:
Freedom Within Confinement

*T*he next six weeks allowed the Jobe Shirt to continue to limit the discomfort and scarring from the healing burn tissue. After the first week of struggling with the garment, Al lessened the time it required to put it on and by the end of the fourth week, he had the routine down to five minutes unaided. The relief he received from the shirt was countered by the pressure that returned to both his eyes. His recovery continued to be a struggle between reprieves from discomfort and immersion back into the abyss of pain.

The scar tissue covering the ducts that drain fluid from the eyes brought unbearable headaches and returned him to the pain of last February. He was given prescriptions of diuretics and painkillers. At his eye examination in early June, Dr. Westmont determined that there were no other options but to operate again. Elaine and Al sat in the examination room as he held up a drawing for Elaine and explained to Al what he would be enduring on the operating table.

"Try to picture an overflowing sink. The drain is clogged

and the water will continue to build unless you find a way to shut off the valve. As the pressure in the eye has continued to build, your eyeball has swollen in size and begun to stretch. The retina attached to the back of the eyeball with rods and cones is not stretching and instead has started to detach from the back of the eye because of its connection to the optic nerve. In essence, we will be shutting off fifty percent of the flow by freezing the gland. We need to operate this afternoon if that works logistically for the two of you."

Elaine and Al had prepared themselves for this possibility, and Al finally broke the silence. "Let's get it over with." The effort to speak reverberated in his head.

Elaine found herself sitting again in the unforgiving orange waiting room chair of Overlook Hospital. Unknown to Al, she had just found out she was pregnant. He had been so overwhelmed with pain that she wanted to wait until he was feeling better to tell him. She ran a hand over her stomach, thought about her surprise and how different, yet the same, the circumstances of today were. She sat waiting for news of her husband, pregnant, but this time with hope.

Please let him keep his eyes. It's what he wants.

Four hours later, Elaine was summoned by the doctor. Al was awake after the surgery, had immediate relief from the intense pain and was asking for her. She followed the doctor down a long wide hallway to the recovery area and Al's bedside.

"Al, I'm here. How do you feel?" Elaine stood at the side of Al's hospital bed that had been wheeled into a recovery room he would be sharing with two other patients.

The haze from the anesthesia clung to him as he tried to focus on Elaine's voice. "I don't feel any pain."

The tension Elaine had felt in her body released its grip. "Al, I think the surgery was a success." The lines of stress and the tense muscles of his were gone.

The haze from the anesthesia continued to loosen its hold on his senses, and he breathed out deeply. "Elaine, I'm free." For the first time since the accident, Al said those words with sincerity.

(212)

"Limited itching, no pain. I'm really free."

Elaine held her hand to her stomach. "We've turned a corner. We've really turned a corner."

"Elaine, this is it. We're getting back to close to a normal life." Al's mind began to clear.

She caught her breath before continuing. "Al, there's more to our new normal. We're having another baby." She squeezed his hand as she spoke.

Al yawned widely. "Wait, what did you say?"

She smiled with tears starting in her eyes. "You heard me. I'm pregnant."

Al smiled broadly. "It didn't beat us. God, I love you. We're a family. Please, I want you to stay home for the next three days, not driving back and forth to the hospital."

Elaine felt giddy. "Maybe I'll have Dad pick you up."

"That's a good idea. Wow." Both Al and Elaine were quiet. "Go home. I'm fine."

"I love you. I'll call tomorrow." Elaine dropped a quick kiss lightly on his lips and unceremoniously left.

Al became fully awake and lay in the quiet of his shared hospital room thinking about the future.

We have a future we are still building. It didn't beat us.

He spent three days in the hospital adapting to a world without pain. On his first day home he was charged with an energy he hadn't felt since before the accident. All he could think about was helping Elaine and bringing their relationship back to the equality it had before October 1.

Elaine stopped him on his way through the kitchen. "I'm getting a bag together for Albert. Your Mom and Fenna are going to watch him this afternoon for us." She kissed Al and then continued moving between the kitchen, nursery, and living room. "Why don't you relax. You shouldn't be so physically active yet." She spoke with distraction as she finished loading a separate bag of food for the toddler.

"I will, but first I'm taking a shower. I don't need to relax." He disappeared while Elaine continued to get Albert ready.

Al came out of the bathroom an hour later looking refreshed. "Dad? Are you still here?"

Mr. Hinds called back to Al from the kitchen. "Fenna and your mom haven't gotten here yet." Mr. Hinds had taken the day off to pick Al up from the hospital and was in no hurry to go home.

Without the aid of his cane, Al found his way to the refrigerator and fished around for the cold cuts he knew would be in the drawer on the left. "I rested for three days. I'm starved for real food and a real life. When is Fenna coming to pick up Albert?" He found the plastic Tupperware container Elaine kept the cold cuts in, grabbed the mustard off the refrigerator door, kicked the door shut with his foot, and turned to the counter where the bread box sat. "Dad, do you want a sandwich?"

Mr. Hinds stretched and relaxed. "Nah, your mother-in-law left lunch for me before she went to work."

It sank into Al that while he fought to get past his world of pain and discomfort, the outside world had to continue with its business. He thought he understood that, but the fact that he was finally about to be a part of it made the possibility real.

He slapped together the sandwich and then spoke between bites. "Now that I'm feeling better Elaine and I can start talking about when I can do some kind of work to bring in a paycheck."

Elaine walked into the kitchen with Albert perched on her hip. "Al, I know you're feeling 100 percent better, but please take it easy. We can kick back and enjoy our afternoon alone together before we start planning to attack the world."

Al thought of their new baby. "Well, not completely alone."

Elaine stopped what she was doing. "Yes. This time next year we'll have two." She knew Al was concerned about her health. "Al, stop worrying. This baby and I will be fine. I didn't feel right with the last pregnancy before you had the accident. It wasn't meant to be."

The sound of a car horn came from the driveway.

"I think your grandma, Aunt Fenna, Steven, and Cheryl are here." Al sat back and prepared for the family assault.

The two cousins squealed with delight, as Steven bolted up

the steps ahead of his mom and grandmom with Cheryl perched on her own mother's hip. "Are you ready for a fun afternoon at Aunt Fenna's?" Albert immediately squirmed out of his mother's arms.

Fenna and Rose Plevier spoke together. "Hi, Al. How are you feeling?"

Al took another bite of the sandwich and spoke around the food. "Normal."

Fenna laughed at the return of her brother's personality. "I can see that."

"I can think." Al wiped his mouth with a napkin.

"Thank you for picking up the little guy today. I may just take a walk with my wife and enjoy the fresh air." Al smiled as he heard the two boys running in circles around the house.

Rose Plevier walked up next to her son. "Don't forget you just got out of the hospital. You deserve time together that isn't measured by doctor's appointments and lifesaving procedures, but don't overdo it." She held out her arms as Cheryl reached to her from Fenna. "Fenna can make dinner while I watch the kids. Albert may be looking for a change of scenery." She smiled at the two boys roughhousing in the living room.

Cheryl babbled into her grandmother's face while Al laughed at the joyful noise he heard. "I guess she agrees that this day works out for everyone. Remember to give Albert back. My family will all be under the same roof tonight sleeping peacefully and soundly."

Chapter XVII: Hubris

"*You* could always do the laundry." Elaine's response to Al's offer of help a week after being home from his procedure was meant as a joke.

"Fine." He shrugged his shoulders and walked out the back door toward the exterior basement stairs that led to the laundry room.

Elaine called loudly after his retreating back. "I was just kidding."

"I'm serious," Al said under his breath to Elaine.

Elaine yelled one last time to him through the open kitchen window. "Great. The laundry room is overflowing, knock yourself out."

Al called over his shoulder. "You shouldn't do any lifting." He walked out the door, down the stairs to the left of the back door and into the laundry room. He found the basket containing his clothes that Elaine had brought down yesterday, where it always sat separately from the other clothes for easy sorting and pinning.

I'll start with mine. I have three loads here anyway. He started to do the one chore he always hated. *What did I get myself into?* He continued with the process and thought about how heavy these baskets must be for Elaine. *I will carry the laundry baskets*

(216)

down here for her. Tomorrow I'll do her laundry, but for today I can get away with washing my clothes and Alberts.

He started to fill the washer, reached for the powder detergent he knew she kept on the shelf to his right, measured what he thought he needed in the plastic cup and tipped it too fast spilling its' contents everywhere. *Shit.* He started to clean up the mess. *I'll put what's in the cup in the washer, get the laundry started and think about cleaning the mess up later.* He continued with the first load and never heard Elaine come up behind him over the sound of the filling washer.

"Al, what are you doing?" She stifled a laugh at the sight of laundry powder all over the front of the washer.

Al was embarrassed and defensive about his latest attempt to help around the house. "I can handle this for the next six months. You can't bring these heavy baskets down here." Al picked up his basket of clothes, shoved some in the washer, and slammed the lid.

Elaine started to bend over to help clean up the mess and then stopped herself. "Now that you volunteered, you can help handle the laundry for the rest of our marriage." She turned laughing and tried to exit quickly. "I have to get out of here before I change my mind."

Al followed his wife out the basement door and then up the stairs next to the kitchen door. "Can you grab my cane for me? I left it next to the back door and I want to go for a walk and start to map out the neighborhood for myself. Care to join me?"

"You told me to relax, remember?" Elaine smiled and walked the four steps inside the kitchen door to get his cane. "Here."

Al felt the cane tap his right hand and he grabbed at it. "I'll be back in a little while. I need to take my time. I'll be doing this by memory." He moved toward the driveway with purpose. *I need some fresh air. She may not care if I get lost for a few hours.* He counted his steps to the edge of the driveway. *I know my way around every inch of this property and to the road. I'll pick up the pace and go a little farther today.* Al walked down the gravel at

(217)

a brisk pace and met the edge of the road in exactly the number of steps he should. *I'll go down and make a right at the end of Lake Road. That should give me a good two to three-mile walk.*

He made the right onto North Road and lost himself in his thoughts. He made another turn onto what he thought was an adjacent road confident at his continued pace and walked straight into a hard, solid object under which his cane had gone.

"Oww! Whoa, where am I?" Al touched his nose and mouth and then reached out and felt the obstacle in front of him. *This is wood, so I am either at the side of a house or, wait a minute. This is a garage door. I better get out of here.*

A female voice spoke out to Al's left side. "Hello? Is someone out there?"

Al didn't know what to say. "Yes, excuse me, but I ran into your garage door." He assumed that the woman had come down and could see his goggles and still bandage eyes from the most recent surgery.

"Al?"

"I guess my reputation precedes me."

Laughing, the woman walked closer to him. "Elaine's probably wondering where you are.

"Actually, I'm wondering where I am." Al scratched his head as he talked.

"You're probably so glad to be home and didn't count your steps." The woman smiled and looked for a reaction from Al.

Which house am I at? I didn't go that far. "I'm ashamed to admit that you're right." Al shifted nervously in front of the woman whose voice he did not recognize.

"Would you like a ride home or do you want to start from scratch and count your steps back?" The woman had seen Al walking before and didn't want to hinder his independence. "Sorry, the garage door was halfway up. We were trying to air it out on such a warm day."

"You should think about that. You never know when a blind guy is going to come by." Al rubbed his nose where he had made contact with the door. "Maybe I'll take that ride home. I can go out with Elaine later and figure out what I did wrong."

The woman looked at Al with admiration. "I have to pull the door the rest of the way up, so you should step back a few more feet." She opened the garage door, slipped behind the wheel of her car and pulled up next to him. "Hop in."

It took every ounce of self-restraint Al had, not to flinch when the car pulled next to him. He opened the door, ducked his head to avoid where he thought the roof was and climbed in. "What kind of car is this? It sounds good."

"Mustang Convertible. Didn't you notice the top was down?" The woman pulled away from the house.

"No, but I feel it now. This is a nice ride." Al remarked with an appreciative smile.

"When was the last time you were in a convertible?" The woman asked innocently.

October 1, 1974, 8:00 o'clock in the morning on a beautiful day like today. "It's been a while." A few minutes later, Al was deposited at his kitchen door. "Thanks. I really appreciate it."

"Tell Elaine, Marybeth said hi." The woman looked at the back door of their house as she spoke.

"Sure. Thanks, Marybeth. I hope I didn't scare you." He stepped back to let her pull out of the driveway.

Mental note: Marybeth lives after the right turn onto North Road. The car pulled away, Al swung his cane and walk down into the basement. He stood in front of the washing machine and heard tires on the driveway. *I'll hide down here as long as I can. I'm not in the mood to talk.*

While he changed the loads in the washer, he heard over his head muffled voices, lots of tiny running feet and then adult footsteps moving across the kitchen and out the back door.

"Al?" Fenna was surprised he was in the basement doing laundry, a chore he hated, so soon after eye surgery. "I'm taking Albert to play with Stephen. Why don't you come up and forget about the laundry?" She waited for him to answer. "Maybe you and Elaine could hire someone to help with the house. You both deserve a break."

Al walked toward her voice. "Thanks, but I don't need help and besides, that costs money." He heard toddling steps over his head and the muffled sound of a baby's voice. He followed Fenna back up the stairs and into the kitchen where he was greeted by happy, running children.

Elaine looked up from packing a bag for Albert and was surprised to see the damage to his nose. "What happened to your face?"

Al touched his nose and forehead. "I met one of the neighbors, the hard way. I walked into some woman named Marybeth's half-open garage door. Nice lady."

Fenna and Elaine looked at each other, shrugged and then both started to gather the three kids, so Albert could have another afternoon with his cousins. "Al, this little guy will see you later. Enjoy dinner tonight. I'll drop off Mom and Albert at six o'clock. You can stay out as late as you like." Fenna had picked up her daughter while Elaine corralled the boys toward the door.

Al tried to stay out of the way of the stampede. "Are we going somewhere tonight?" He absentmindedly rubbed his forehead.

Elaine looked at the growing red mark. "You want ice for your face?"

"Nah." Al heard the happy feet of the two boys running. "You have fun today with your cousins, big guy."

Fenna loaded the kids into her car and pulled away beeping the horn. Elaine came in to find Al reaching into the cookie jar. "Try not to fill up." She needed tonight out with friends so she and Al could start feeling like a couple.

He replaced the lid on the cookie jar. "Where we going?"

"We're having dinner with the Lisandro's, remember?"

"Not at all. Let's get ready before I change my mind." Al reached back into the jar and grabbed two more cookies. "Did you tell them I still have my bandages?"

"Al, the Lisandro's are both blind. It's a chance for us to get out in a relaxed environment while you're recovering. I told them how well the surgery went."

(220)

The blind couple Elaine and Al had befriended before the accident, Audrey and Rich Lisandro, thought dinner together in a semi-formal atmosphere was a great opportunity for Al to learn from them as he acclimated back into a social life. They prepared the dinner and asked only that Elaine relax.

An hour after arriving at the Lisandro's, Elaine found herself leaving behind some of the stress of the last eight months as the conversation continued with ease. While the couples enjoyed dessert and coffee no one knew the sun was setting except Elaine. It was a clear warm night and Elaine did not think to mention this fact, because she was still able to see in the darkening house at 8 o'clock on the warm June evening. The sun was very low and the room was growing steadily darker.

"Have you two decided on a name for the baby?' Audrey directed the question to Elaine.

"Either Lawrence, after my father, or Pamela, if it's a girl." Elaine finished and reached carefully across the table.

"That's sweet. Your dad must be thrilled." Audrey sipped her coffee before she continued. "I was glad to hear that you could come over tonight." Audrey added milk to her coffee, discretely inserting the tip of her forefinger into the cup.

Al jumped in. "I'm actually feeling fine. Much better than before I went in. I hope this procedure lasts longer than the last one. The next surgery I hope to have is for the corneal transplant." He sat back in the chair and relaxed.

"Wouldn't that be perfect to have the transplant right before the baby is born?" Rich, living with a permanent loss of his sight, envied his friend's potential good luck.

"That would be great, but I don't want to get my hopes up. As long as the baby is healthy, I'll worry about me later." Al took a sip of his coffee. "Elaine, could you pass the milk please?"

With the guidance of the shadows, Elaine sat trying to remember where she last saw the creamer. She heard Audrey pouring something and assumed now that it was near her. "Audrey, could you pass the milk to me?"

"Oh, sorry Elaine." Al, aware of where Audrey was sitting,

stood slightly and held his right hand above the table.

"Here you go, Al. Which hand do you have out? Audrey extended her right hand in front of her as she also stood.

Elaine watched the shadowy figures maneuver and recognized the analogy Al discussed with her after he lost his sight. He believed living without sight was an obstacle that could be overcome with the mechanics of procedure and methodology. At times, he told her, it was nothing more than a 'pain-in-the-ass'.

The two exchanged the creamer and returned to their seats. "Even with the practice I've had with life skills, I got lost today in my own neighborhood." He waited for the shocked surprise from his dinner companions.

"Get used to it. Your cane is your best friend, and it is controlled by a mind that has to constantly stay alert." Rich laughed remembering his own experiences.

Al laughed at the incident. "I thought I had the neighborhood memorized."

Audrey smiled across the table. "Elaine, how long was it before you knew he was gone?"

Having finished her piece of cake, Elaine carefully reached in front of her across the darkened table for her glass of milk. "I never knew."

"Al, did you miscount your steps?" Audrey carefully and quietly placed her empty cup on the saucer in front of her.

"Today I think my failure was a little cockiness and getting caught up in the nice weather. The next thing I knew, I ran face first into the half opened, pull up garage door of a woman I'd never met before. Thank God, my wife knows everyone, because this woman didn't try to shoot me." Al reached under the table and grabbed Elaine's knee.

"That was Marybeth Martinson. I stop to chat with her on my walks with the baby." Elaine drained her milk glass.

Al laughed as the two couples finished the first round of coffee. "I think she thought I was going to rob her."

"I'm sure you present a scary picture." Audrey pushed herself away from the table and rose out of her chair. "Who would like ice cream?"

"That sounds good." Al continued to lean back in his chair.

"Elaine, would you like to come with me?" Audrey confidently walked into the kitchen.

It was now 8:30 and the house was cloaked is semi-dark. "Sure." *This should be interesting. I don't want them to know the lights are out yet. I can still see, more or less. I should try to use the bathroom and see how that works out before I leave.*

Al continued his conversation. "I loved your cake, but my appetite is nonstop lately."

Elaine felt along the back of the dining room chairs as she focused on keeping up with Audrey. "Thank goodness for that. He was beginning to scare me back in January."

"She's right. My weight was around 135 and dropping fast. I had no interest in eating." Al listened to Elaine working her way across the dining room. "Elaine, you sound like you're having trouble walking. Is your back bothering you?" He recalled how Elaine complained about her back during her pregnancy with Little Albert in the first trimester.

"No. I'm a little stiff." She found her way to the other side of the table, counted two chairs and then, putting her hands out in front of her, felt for the swinging door that led to the kitchen. She was not sure where to go, so she stood at the doorway waiting for a cue. "Audrey, do you need help?"

"No, I have it. I thought you might want to get up and move around." Audrey adeptly found the ice cream in the freezer and spooned it into one of the waiting bowls on the counter. "I should have served this after dinner and before the cake, but I forgot."

"Your black forest cake was delicious." Elaine could see clearly while the freezer door was open and the light inside shone brightly but she did not want to cheat so she waited for Audrey to close the door.

"Thank you, I love to cook and bake. I'd like to think I'm pretty good at it after all these years." Audrey picked up the bowl

(223)

and began to walk toward Elaine.

"No, thank you. I had two servings of the cake and that's more than usual." She began to back out of the kitchen, felt her back softly meet the door, and pushed it open, holding it wide for Audrey to pass through.

"You can go ahead." Audrey appreciated Elaine's courtesy, but silently thought this was as good a time as any to prove a blind person's independence, even on such a small scale.

Elaine turned to her left and felt the china cabinet. It was getting close to 9 o'clock and the heavily treed yard of the blind couple had added to the darkness. Knowing she was past the back of Rich's chair, she took one step to her right and felt for the two chairs next to Rich on his side of the table. She reached the last chair on that side and walked around it to her side of the table. She found her chair, pulled it out slightly and slid gratefully onto the padded seat.

After another hour of lingering conversation, Al turned to Elaine. "We should get going."

"It was fun to have you over. We have to do this again soon." Audrey rose from the table in unison with her guests and husband.

Elaine put her arm through Al's. "Elaine, I have my cane, you don't need to lead me."

"Actually, you're leading me." She still did not mention that the four of them sat in total darkness, preferring to let him believe she was being romantic.

As Al and Elaine were leaving, Audrey reached for the outside light switch out of courtesy to Elaine and felt the one next to it in the off position. "Elaine, did you turn on any of the lamps?"

"No." She knew her secret was out and smiled at her friend's surprise.

"But this switch is off. Have you been sitting in the dark throughout dinner?" She was overcome with embarrassment and guilt.

"I wanted to experience life from all of your perspectives. I haven't had the time to do that during these past eight months. In the last two hours, I had a sample of the frustration and patience involved living without sight." The explanation was simple for such a large gesture.

Al had never considered asking Elaine to try something like this. He was speechless and broke the moment with sarcasm. "You gain that ability by being married."

Elaine squeezed her husband's arm. "Thank you for dinner. It was delicious and interesting." She let go of Al and hugged both Rich and Audrey.

Al and Elaine walked hand in hand to the car. At the passenger side door, he put his hand behind her neck and kissed her thoroughly before climbing into the passenger seat. "I love you."

She kissed him back and smiled with satisfaction. "Me too. Let's go home."

Chapter XVIII: Journeys

A week later, on their anniversary June 19, Elaine had another chance to view life from Al's perspective. He had begun to do more extensive chores around the house including replacing light fixtures. Relying on the skills he had learned in the building trades, he compensated for his loss of sight as he worked on the electricity in their refurbished home.

The electrical work was not an impossible task for a man without sight, but it quadrupled the time required to finish the task. He was able to shut off the main power to the house and then feel the wires on the project on which he was working. The main requirement was to have someone else first point out the white, black and grounding wire colors, and then stand by as he marked them with tapes or twist ties to differentiate them.

As he worked diligently that day, he didn't realize how much time had passed as he changed out the light fixture to save the expense of an electrician. The summer day had been warm and Elaine enjoyed the air passing through the open windows that refreshed the house.

It grew later until finally, the sun began to set. Elaine put Albert to sleep for the night at eight o'clock and wondered what was taking Al so long. *He hasn't even asked me what time it is.* She tiptoed out of the nursery immersed in the darkness of the house. *I might as well see what it's like to live in his world at home. At least until he yells for dinner.*

As the last shadow left the house, Elaine made her way across the living room continuously stubbing her toes on toys strewn across the floor. In the kitchen, she could hear Al working on his project with the occasional obligatory swearing and toss of a tool.

As she reached the screen back door, she yelled out the door toward the basement staircase and the open door at the bottom. "Al, I'm getting something to eat. Do you want anything?"

"Let me finish up. I'll be done in a few minutes." The sound of more tools hitting the floor could be heard. "There goes another tool into never, never land. That's it, Elaine. I've decided if I drop something, it's gone forever unless somebody with sight finds it."

I'll make a note of that. Elaine kept her thoughts to herself. *I'm starving. I hope I don't look like a house by the time this baby is born. I'll give the kitchen a try in the dark and see what happens.* She traveled around the kitchen by memory, trying to count drawers and feeling for utensils. *Moonlight does not even penetrate the windows with all the trees on our property. I never noticed that before. It's so dark here even on a clear night. Let me see if I can figure out which food is which in the fridge.*

"Elaine, the electricity is on." Al walked in the back door slamming the screen behind him. "What's for dinner?"

The fridge light flickered on as she opened the door and she was disappointed. *I'm too hungry to leave the lights off.* Her eyes panned over the leftovers from last night. "Leftovers. Did you change the fixtures down there?" She pulled the Tupperware containers out of the fridge and moved toward the cabinets that held the pots.

"Yes. Why did we ever buy a house this old?" He pulled a bar stool with his foot and plopped down on the cushion with exaggeration. "Sorry it took me so long. I dropped my tools a couple of times and spent half an hour crawling on my hands and knees looking for them."

"That'll teach ya." Elaine let the comment hang in the air.

"I don't care why I lose something, but it's the most annoying thing about not having sight. It's even worse when I'm outside and I drop things in the grass. I'm not going to bother trying to find things outside anymore. Whatever I drop is gone." Al got up, walked over to the fridge, grabbed the apple juice, and gave the door a slam.

"You always seem to find my tea mug." Elaine took a pot from the cabinet as the mental image of Al constantly knocking over her mugs flashed.

Al flipped on the radio. An unknown station blared back at him. "You changed my station. We need new rules." He fooled around with the dial and then finally gave up. "Second most annoying thing; finding a radio station."

"You are on a tear tonight. What's bugging you?" Elaine finished heating up the leftovers and let them simmer.

"Money and the lawsuit. So much paperwork and for what?" Al banged his hand on the counter.

"Have you been thinking about money the whole time you were working on the electric?" Elaine took two plates from the cabinet. "Please get our drinks, Sweetheart."

"I already got juice." He took a long sip straight out of the container and burped. "Excuse me."

Elaine turned to face her husband. "I'm glad you're satisfied, now get me a drink. I'll have something for you to eat in a minute or so."

What's her problem? I spent half the day on the electric and now she's snippy.

Al walked over to the fridge, appeased Elaine with the milk container and went back to the subject that was foremost in his mind. "We were starting to build our nest egg and now we have

(228)

to start over. Neither one of us cared if we both worked or when I had to work two jobs. We didn't ask anybody for anything and now, we have to fight to keep our heads above water. I'm tired of it already."

Elaine looked over at him with a concentrated and worried gaze. "What's wrong? Are your headaches coming back?"

"No." He let out a long breath. "I'm tired, I guess." Al took another sip from the almost empty container and became quiet as recognition and guilt entered his self-centered rant. "Oooops." Al held the juice container in front of his face, mid-thought, as the revelation of a forgotten milestone jumped into his head. "I'm so sorry. I forgot our anniversary." For the first time in their four-year marriage, he had not given it a thought. "A couple of light fixtures in the laundry room isn't what I would have had in mind for a gift if I had remembered on time." He put down the container and started to wring his hands.

Elaine suddenly felt bad for him. "Money is tight for us. What I really want is a day off. Let's send the baby over to my mother's and you can wait on me all day." She spooned out the leftovers and brought a plate to Al. "She mentioned to me yesterday that she would like to give us a day off as an anniversary gift."

"That works. Wouldn't you like a gift too?" Al hung his head down as his mood worsened. "Forgetting an anniversary is something that's supposed to happen after ten or twenty years together. I'm sorry, Honey."

She tried not to laugh at the sullen expression on his face. "I forgive you."

He felt recharged. "How do I know that you didn't just remember?"

"Trust me, I didn't forget." She placed her hands over his across the counter.

"Fine. Call your mom tomorrow and see if she and dad can watch Albert on Saturday. We can order pizza and stay in bed all day." Al started to envision a day for both of them.

"That sounds great." Elaine began to eat dinner.

(229)

Al ate almost all his meatloaf before he continued. "The money has been bothering me all day. Can we go over our situation now? If I don't, I'll be up all night."

"Why don't we do it after dinner? We can go over the finances and discuss our options on a full stomach before you become too aggravated." She took another bite and swallowed before continuing. "No looking back, only forward."

"Do you realize what you would be doing right now if it wasn't for the accident and our loss of income?" Al dropped his fork on his plate. "You'd be living in Rainbow Lake and looking for a summer house at the shore," Al spoke with disgust.

"That's what's bothering you? A house at the shore? Are you serious?" Elaine shook her head and squeezed her eyes shut in anger.

"No, it's not that." Al stopped when he realized how materialistic he sounded. "I don't know. I feel that was what we should have and now we don't. Are we always going to be starting over? I'm tired." He held his hand to his head.

"You're out of the hospital after your third stay in a year, and because you finally are living without discomfort you want to take on the world?" She took a sip of her milk and looked over at the almost empty cookie jar with hunger beginning to overwhelm her. "We'd have more money, so what? We'll always make money and we'll always have to work for it. Thank God, we had our investment properties and a little money put away before the accident. Imagine what life would be like if we didn't have that. At least we'll have a chance to rebuild our finances and our lives as a family. Would you rather be dead and have Albert and I living off your life insurance without you? How would life be for him to grow up without his father?" Elaine knew she opened up an old wound, but felt this might bring clarity to the dark future he was envisioning.

He held up his hands in surrender. "I got it, take it easy." He heard her take a side step away from the counter. "Are you going after the cookies?"

"Do you have a comment about that too?" Elaine held up a

(230)

cookie in midair challenging him.

He put his hands up in a gesture of surrender. "No, it's all good. Eat up."

She took a large bite and walked back to the counter. "Mr. Bayplaza wants to talk to us sometime this week. He said we don't have to come to the office, we can talk on the phone. I didn't want to bother you before the surgery, but since you need a battle to fight, do it with a lawyer." She finished her cookie and then reached to the cabinet on her left for the refill bag. "Where's my stash?"

Al felt himself trying to blend into the counter. "The cookies are in my tool belt. I took them earlier." He felt the daggers Elaine shot as silence fell over the two of them. "There's about half a bag left."

"Go get them. No wonder you weren't hungry for dinner." She stood on the other side of the counter.

"Relax." Al rose dutifully and reached around the back of the chair and pulled the bag of cookies from his tool belt and handed it over.

She grabbed the bag from his still moving hand. "Thanks."

After cleaning up the dinner dishes, the two to them sat down and began to sort bills, statements, and accounts that represented the agony of medical problems and procedures.

"How do you want to start?" Elaine plowed ahead before he could answer. "The South Amboy house is still on the market, but we haven't had any reasonable offers. Real estate is soft right now, but it makes more sense to sell it, rather than collect the little bit of rent we are getting that barely covers the mortgage and taxes. The house made sense when it was an investment that paid for itself, but we need the cash out of the place."

"After the mortgage is paid, how do we stand?" Al had to admit he had no idea what the balance was on the mortgage anymore.

"If we lower our asking price, it will barely cover it. We have to stay firm a little longer. Lou lowered his commission to help us out." The mention of Lou, the real estate agent that worked with Al on all his real estate deals in the past, brought a sense of nostalgia to the stark numbers that now sat before them.

"That was nice of him. We should stay firm on the price as long as we can. Do you have the book of the house expenses for this place?" Al folded and unfolded his hands in front of him.

"With taxes, mortgage, electric, oil, food, car insurance, house insurance, and gas for the car, we need about $800.00 a month just to survive. That does not include car repairs, house repairs or miscellaneous items figured in." Elaine lifted the adding machine she brought from the kitchen.

"You mean like a catastrophic accident?" Al rubbed his stomach and felt the leftovers lie like a rock at the bottom.

"Al, let's go forward with this." Elaine reached for one particular pile of statements. "This should make you feel good. I'll tell you what the medical expenses have been up to now. All of them are covered, but that should give you an idea of what we would have faced without Worker's Compensation." She held the statements in front of her. "The first hospital stay was $28,000. The total bills that I have received statements for are $40,000."

Al blew a low whistle and stopped. "We could never have paid that." He dropped his hands down in front of him. "We need money." The dead statement of fact rallied him.

"The disability check is $448.00 per month. We also have our savings, so using subtraction I'd say we can live off that and the kindness of our families for about twelve more months." Elaine pulled the file for the South Amboy house toward her. "If the money from the sale of the Amboy house is what we are asking, or say we get $5000 less, that would give us $4000 in liquidity, which included the original deposit and a little more breathing time of about eleven to twelve months including the disability money. That breathing time is only for our basic needs."

"We need money," Al repeated the thought foremost in his mind. "There has to be a way for me to work." His mind raced as he thought about jobs that did not require sight.

"Al, you're only allowed to earn a certain amount of money working or you'll lose the disability. I have the form for that here in your Worker's Comp file." Elaine sorted papers as Al sat in amazement at how organized Elaine had become in spite of the time she spent taking care of him and Albert.

"Al, we should double check these figures, but what I have written down is that you can only earn $4,200 a year working or you will lose your benefits." She stopped to see her husband's reaction.

"Mr. Bayplaza explained that to me and it still doesn't make any sense. We need around $9,600 a year to live comfortably with some kind of a cushion and not live spoon to mouth. I could probably pick up work through the Blind Commission for around $2,000 to $3,000 a year, but that would still leave us with the need to supplement $2,800 a year after Workers' Comp. If you start working we wouldn't even need that, but damn it, I paid into that and I should receive something. I don't think I can pull off the $9,600 alone right now. I'll ask Mr. Bayplaza." Al put his hands to his forehead in a gesture he always used when he was thinking hard for a solution.

"We still have the outcome of the case as an option." Elaine stopped sifting the papers in front of her and looked at her husband.

"That's not an option, it's the Irish Sweepstakes. I'm not even going to figure that into our options at this juncture." Al did not try to hide the disgust in his voice.

"Mr. Bayplaza never said it would be easy fighting a third-party lawsuit, but he does think we have a good chance to settle. It will take time and patience." Elaine went back to the subject of her return to the workforce. "I can teach again. You know how much I loved it, but let's concentrate on getting you healthy enough to stay home and take care of the kids. To be honest, I have looked into the availability of teaching positions since January in my old district and through various contacts. There's nothing available right now." She waited a few seconds as she pretended to look through papers before continuing.

Al sat still. "Wow. Things are tight. Are there not enough jobs or too many people to fill them?"

"Both." The role reversal that had taken place with Al and Elaine loomed large in front of him.

"If you want to work, that's fine. It's obvious we will need the money, but I have to contribute more to this marriage than as a babysitter."

"It's not babysitting. It's raising our children." Now it was Elaine's turn to grow angry. "One of us has to be home or the kids will be shipped to a babysitter."

"I understand that, but I still have to contribute something to support this family." His mind began to race as he thought about possible jobs he could do to support them until he could start a small business out of the house. "I could do phone sales while the kids are asleep, and Kindergarten is only five years away for the new baby."

Al took his hands away from his forehead and clasped them in front of him as he continued. "The phone sales could carry us through until I can find the cash to seed a small service business and a relative to manage it."

"We have to come up with the seed money first." Elaine didn't want to destroy her husband's sense of self. "We need to start where we are today. I think a small business would be the way we will have to go, but we cannot jump into that now. The disability is your contribution until we figure out another source." Elaine saw a defeated look on Al's face and quickly continued her monologue. "Al, it was the money you earned working two jobs that purchased the Amboy house and this one. I was able to stay home with Albert while you worked. Believe me, I'm not worried about your ability to generate income, I don't want you to consider that now."

He bent his head down toward his folded hands. "I got it. I know what you're thinking and I agree. Having bills hanging over our heads without a concrete plan for paying them and losing the chance to live a good life isn't a lifestyle I can maintain."

(234)

"Find out about telemarketing jobs for the both of us. I can start it with you and after the baby is born, I will send my resume out and start looking for a teaching position." Elaine put the papers back into the manila folders and stared at her inventory of paperwork.

"I'll get on it tomorrow morning." He felt he had gained control or at least partial control over their lives. "Baby, I'm starting to think we're going to work our way back to our old life. As long as I'm feeling good, I can work toward doing more than floating our financial boat."

"Are you ready to relax?" She turned away from the mountain in front of her and looked at her husband sitting safely next to her.

"Our lives are so unpredictable." He placed his hands flat on the table in front of him. "We expected that our lives would be more or less like our parents as we raised our family and built our nest egg, but it was all an illusion. It was gone in an instant without any control or choice." Al shook his head, pushed himself away from the table and walked toward their bedroom anticipating the oblivion of sleep after a large dinner and long day of work.

That night he dreamed in vivid colors and details of a beach with white sand and a brilliant blue sky and a few fluffy white clouds. On the beach were Elaine and Albert, but it wasn't a beach in New Jersey, it was in Jamaica, from their honeymoon. The trip to Jamaica was the only time he had ever traveled outside the tristate area. He found joy in traveling and was eager to go somewhere distant.

The ocean in the dream had different hues of blue that were a stark and beautiful contrast to the gray-blue of the New Jersey Atlantic he was used to. A breeze that he could not feel warmed by the bright yellow sunshine, played softly over Elaine's hair and drew his attention to the sound of moving lush, deep green palms behind him. As the palms moved, brown palms ready to fall were visible giving up the secret of the coconuts that lay beneath them. He heard Elaine's laughter as he saw her holding their son.

Elaine appeared young in the dream as she looked on their

honeymoon, carefree and in love. She held Albert high up in the air as he screamed with joy. Albert was a baby, not yet a toddler, with chubby cheeks and two bottom teeth. Al walked over to his family, and Elaine brought the baby down to hold between the two of them. Over her swimsuit, she wore a wrap made of gauzy fabric with a flowered pattern blending many hues of blue to match her eyes. The two of them were laughing, holding hands, and he grew confused as to why Albert was with them in Jamaica. He looked at Elaine's face and thought she should look a few years older with short blond hair. He looked toward the sky and decided to forget his questions until he felt the heat of the sun in his dream and worried that it was not good for his burns. It was then that he abruptly awakened.

She looked like she had the last day I left for work. I should have known it was a dream. I'll never see her change. Albert will always be a baby in my mind's eye. I can feel him with my hands, but never watch him grow. I'll always dream about the past.

Elaine heard her husband call her name in his dream and then felt his body awaken with a shake. "Al?"

"I'm sorry, did I wake you?" He reached under the covers and touched her.

"It sounded like you were having a nightmare." She adjusted her pillow and rolled to her side.

"No, I didn't have a nightmare." *I'm living a nightmare.*

Elaine rolled over and fell quickly back to sleep. Al lay awake for the rest of the night trying to make sense of his circumstances and rose the next morning earlier than Elaine and Albert. By the time Mr. Bayplaza phoned to discuss the status of the lawsuit, Al was anxious and exhausted.

His worry was apparent. "How is our position?"

The lawyer never wasted time with small talk. "We started with nine companies including A&K and their mother company, Oka, Oka, and Eunvea."

"I thought we couldn't sue A&K?" The mention of his former employer brought a tightness to his chest.

(236)

"Remember what I told you in February? We are trying to position one company against the other. The suit against A&K was dismissed without merit, but the company did willingly open the files with the necessary information I needed to move forward. Our three main targets now are MTZW who made the shower head, McClintock Plastic who made the tubing, and BBLvd who made the protective boots and is the mother company for Safety Blvdhtous, the clothing manufacturer. We've created a triangle, and I believe MTZW will be found to be the main target. We will use the other companies for the information that can be provided by them to support our case. You have your disability now, but if you win the lawsuit, the balance that was paid to you will be deducted from the final settlement."

Al laughed derisively. "My wife explained that to me. I can't live off what Worker's Compensation is sending me now, and they're going to add insult to injury by taking it back?"

"If, and that's a big if, the settlement is substantial. New Jersey is one of two states where an employee cannot sue an employer or fellow employees. The state requires a victim to pay back the money collected from Worker's Compensation including the medical from any punitive damages that are awarded." Mr. Bayplaza found himself cut off by Al, a reaction he was not used to and rarely tolerated.

"All I want is a chance to have my life back. Isn't it bad enough that I may never see?" Residual self-pity and anger from last night's discussion enveloped him. He gripped the phone cord, clenched his jaw, and felt a headache starting.

"One thing at a time. If the litigants can make the case that you were 51 percent responsible, you will lose. You can always appeal a case but if you lose, the uphill battle you were fighting would now include pushing a boulder ahead of you. My fee is one -third of the final settlement." He stopped at the last point.

"Let's keep moving." *I know you're worth it, but shit.*

"I have copies of your disability claim in front of me. You have to schedule an appearance and speak before the judge in court. It still has to be determined whether you are temporarily or

(237)

Jayne Kelly

permanently disabled."

Al felt his temperament wearing thin. "Got it."

"Have you made the necessary appointments with the disability doctors? We can't move forward until you do." Mr. Bayplaza looked at the paperwork in front of him as he spoke with Al on the phone. "You have to understand that disability assumes you are incapacitated and cannot work to your full potential. Our lawsuit assumes that your life has been permanently altered in a manner that renders you incapable of supporting your family and that your quality of life has been diminished."

"My life is permanently altered, and I can no longer work as a chemical engineer or do construction to build our future finances." Al took a breath to regain his composure. "I'm not looking for a pot of gold. I'm looking to be a productive part of society. Man, I want to work, pay my bills, and have some kind of future."

Mr. Bayplaza ignored Al's rant. "Did you see any of the disability doctors yet?"

Al's patience was gone and he let his sarcasm invade the conversation. "I saw the Optometrist. He says I'm blind. The shrink thinks I'm a wise ass."

Mr. Bayplaza jumped into Al's second rant. "Don't smart mouth those people. Their opinions are a decisive factor in your case. Don't be stupid."

Al took another breath. "You go to some of the gross offices of these guys. I may not be able to see them but I can smell them." He crinkled his nose at the memory.

"These contractors work for the government." Mr. Bayplaza rolled his eyes and pushed forward. "Is that everyone the caseworker wants you to see?"

"No, I have a doctor to see about the burns." Al stopped moving in the chair where he sat and allowed the Jobe suit to do its job.

"We will settle this. It's going to take years, but we will do it. I have to run. I'll be in touch in a few weeks." Art Bayplaza hung up the phone before Al could ask any more questions.

(238)

Rude, but good. "Elaine?" Al rose from the stool he had been sitting on and went to look for his wife. He heard a voice on the other side of the house respond.

"Yes?" She walked out of the master bedroom still holding the miniature shirt she had been folding.

"You want to take Albert for a walk with me? He might go down for an afternoon nap if we take him out in his stroller." Al wanted to get out of the house and clear his mind. "I'm not ready to walk alone with him yet." Al was willing to try anything but not at expense of his family's safety.

"Let's give it a try. You can tell me what the lawyer said." She tossed Albert's shirt onto a chair and walked into the toddler's new room. "Come on cutie. Do you want to go for a walk with me and daddy? You can bring your new bear."

The toddler protested leaving his spot on the carpet where he had created his own world. "No, no, no."

"Yes, yes, yes. You can play in here later." She picked him up and walked out of the room, past the nursery that waited for the arrival of the new baby.

Al heard the approach of Elaine's shoes. "There you two are. Albert, it's so warm outside that I bet you see lots of bunnies and maybe a deer run across the road." Al waited by the kitchen door for his family.

"Al, it's the middle of the day. We've never seen a deer until after dinner." Elaine walked past him with the baby in her arms and down the steps to the stroller which was always left by the back door in good weather.

Like a two-year-old would know. "Want to go down to the river?" Al needed to get out of his own head.

"Yes." Elaine started to relax into her family time and let Albert get down and climb into the stroller by himself. They walked together in silence down the driveway until

Elaine peeked into the stroller and saw Albert's sleeping form. "That didn't take long."

"Look, a deer!" Al pointed ahead of himself with his cane.

"Where?" Elaine stopped and looked at where Al pointed

with his cane. "Very funny." She grabbed his free hand and pushed the stroller with the other.

Al held his stomach and laughed uncontrollably. "Let me have my moment. That lawyer made me crazy. What can I tell you? I can hear deer hooves thirty feet away."

"Ha, ha." A blue jay swooped down a few feet in front of the couple screeching. "Did you hear that? We must be near its nest." Elaine looked around the surrounding tree tops.

Al finally stopped laughing but continued to smile. "Did I ever tell you about the bet I lost?"

"What are you talking about now?" She laughed with him.

"In High School, I was seeing Kathy Chriseen on and off, so Patti Larabe and I made a bet that if I got the worst grade on a test we were taking, I had to ask you out. I barely passed the test, but I got a new girlfriend." He kissed her firmly.

Elaine grasped his hand tighter. "I guess when JFK High School was built, it shifted school districts and our lives."

Al continued to reminisce. "I never spent any time outside the confines of the state of New Jersey before you came into my life. The district shift opened up all new areas of life for me. I swear sometimes I think that if that hadn't happened, I would still be living in a different house, but on the same block, hanging out at the local watering hole. See what you did for me?"

If it wasn't for me, you wouldn't have gone to college, and maybe you wouldn't have gotten the job at the plant, and maybe you wouldn't be suffering like this. The internal admonishment was verbally unexpressed, but proof of the selfless, unequivocal love Elaine always did and always would have for Al. As her mother told Elaine early in the courtship, 'He's the One'.

"When are you supposed to go to court with Mr. Bayplaza for the disability hearing?" She tried to change thoughts away from ones of misplaced guilt.

Al knew the abrupt change in conversation was more than a bit of information she needed. "What are you upset about? Try not to bring up his name for another hour. My stomach is sour from the whole conversation."

(240)

"I asked if you had a date yet." She pulled her hand back in a defensive gesture.

"Out of nowhere?" He reached for her hand.

Elaine found her voice. "I can't help but wonder, if we hadn't gotten together and I hadn't talked you into going to college instead of working steady construction, maybe this wouldn't have happened to you."

Al shook his head in astonishment. "What wouldn't have happened to me? Marriage, my son, a happy life, a big extended family, a new baby, or the will to live?" Al held her hand tightly and stopped walking, bringing Elaine and the stroller to an abrupt stop. "You saved my life on a thousand different levels. The most obvious one is that if I had not gone to college, I would have been drafted and sent to Nam. I might not have come home from that. The accident happened and that is that. You and the kids make it all bearable. I can't imagine my life without you in it."

She leaned her head on his shoulder and heard Albert stir. "We better keep moving."

Chapter XIX: Give and Take

*T*hree weeks later, Al and his attorney were sitting in a courtroom in Newark New Jersey. Mr. Bayplaza had received notice that the case was to be heard at one o'clock, but he and Al needed to be present and ready to go at nine o'clock. As luck would have it, the court log for that day was rescheduled and their case was presented by ten o'clock. It was July 10, and the east coast inner city building air conditioning was not effective enough to accommodate the crowded courtroom.

Al pulled at the tie the lawyer suggested he wear and complained to himself. *Too bad I didn't lose my sense of smell in the accident. I'm probably the worst offender.*

"How are you doing, Al?" Mr. Bayplaza looked over at his client, who was shifting on the bench.

"Fine, no problem." *If I had to sit here until one o'clock, I'd scream.*

"Plevier?" The bailiff read his name. Al and Mr. Bayplaza rose from their seats and moved toward the front of the room.

The judge looked up from behind a pair of bifocals. "I've read the file, and according to the caseworker, you have visited all the necessary physicians, who have declared you permanently disabled. The judge looked through the book in front of him. "For an individual who has been blinded on the job, the award is $50,000. You are given $.75 per square inch of burned tissue. The $50,000 will be divided over a nine-year period at which point you will be re-evaluated."

"Thank you, Your Honor." Mr. Bayplaza ushered Al out of the courtroom after he had answered some perfunctory questions from the Judge.

In the hallway, Al lost control. "I don't believe this. I can't see. I can't SEE! I have to rethink this. Get me home. This isn't right, I paid into that fund."

"Calm down. This is only the beginning. I told you not to expect much. That Judge works for New Jersey, not for the disabled clients walking through the doors. His job is to give only what the client is legally entitled to. The system is not perfect, but this is all you have to work with right now." Mr. Bayplaza kept ushering Al out of the building and toward the parking lot.

"How am I going to tell my wife? Man, this is unbelievable." Al continued to shake his head as he walked and both men stopped next to the passenger side door of Mr. Bayplaza's car. "What am I going to do?" Al's speech trailed off.

He came home that afternoon to more bad news. The realtor had a buyer with cash for the rental property in South Amboy, but the offer was lower than what it was listed for.

"We're going to walk away from this with $1,000. What do you want to do?" Elaine sat outside with her husband, under an umbrella on the battered lawn furniture.

"Our options are limited. Get rid of it, and let's move forward. At least we know where we stand. No more wondering. We're definitely in financial trouble." He thought hard. "We may have to sell this place since I'm only allowed to make $4,000 a year with the phone sales job."

"If I can find a position, I'll teach now and not wait until the baby is born. I miss it anyway. You know I always planned to go back when the children were older." She looked down, laid one hand on her stomach, and imagined who the new baby would look like.

"We only have six months of savings to feed us and cover bills with the disability money. I don't want to lose this house and start over. We would still have to pay rent somewhere with two kids." Al's expression was growing stone-like.

"Not if we live with my family until the case is resolved and I'm working full time. You could take seed money from the sale of this house and start the service business with Mel." She reached for his hand and felt sweat in his palm. "You're feeling so much better with your Jobe shirt, and we have the new baby coming." Elaine stopped and looked over at Al's strained face. "Let's try to enjoy the summer, live off what we have, and make our final decisions in September. This may be our last summer in our own home for a while if our finances don't improve." Elaine waited for him to interrupt her with a happy interjection. "We're celebrating Albert's birthday next week, and I'm looking forward to having the party outside. He's going to be thrilled with the cake this year. I'm making a small circus train I saw in a party cake book. This year he's old enough to understand. I wonder what he's going to think about all the presents you know our families will shower on him?" Elaine planned on hanging balloons all over the house and on the tree branches outside. "I think he's going to be over the moon about everything." Al was silent, and Elaine waited for him to come out of his gloom. "Al?"

"I'm sorry, Sweetheart." Al was interrupted by the sound of Little Albert.

Grateful for the chance to leave, Elaine stood up. "I'll get him. You stay here and think about my cake."

As the weeks of summer passed, Al and Elaine watched their savings dwindle. The fall season approached and the first anniversary of the accident loomed like a dark shadow. Al had accepted a job telemarketing that added an extra $3,000 a year to the household income, but it was still not enough to keep the house for another year.

He was alone one day when the phone rang. "Hello?"

A young woman's voice spoke with perkiness. "Can I speak to Mr. Plevier?"

Al immediately decided the woman was a telemarketer and spoke gruffly. "What can I do for you?"

The young woman continued with hesitation in her voice. "I'm from the firm of McKelvy and Ryan. We represent the estate of Sheila Greene?"

Al stood by the phone for a minute and then the name began to sound familiar. "I think I did a construction job for her two or three years ago."

The woman continued apprehensively. "She passed away on September 2 and we are probating her will. She thought very highly of you and left a small check for you and your family." The secretary waited for a response from Al. "Mr. Plevier?"

He shook himself out of his stunned silence. "Yes, I'm still here. Did she know I got hurt?"

The small home construction job and the extra work he had done at no charge for the elderly woman came back to him. He remembered how kind and helpless she had seemed with nobody to take care of the house with her. She had asked if he could fix the front door in addition to the work he was hired to do and when she tried to pay him, he declined. The elderly woman mentioned how much safer she felt with the extra locks he had added to secure the door.

The young woman now began to talk quickly. "I'm not sure. We don't have that information, but we would like to know when you could come by the office, sign for and pick up the check?" The secretary sounded busy and eager to be off the phone. "I'm sorry, I have someone in the waiting area."

Al did not hesitate. "Tomorrow. I need the phone number and address." He moved over to the typewriter he kept permanently on the counter since it had become increasingly impossible for Elaine to read some of his writing. "Go ahead." He typed the address, phone number, and the time of the appointment.

"Are you in an office? I hear a typewriter." The secretary Thought she had called a home number.

"No, I'm blind and I'm putting this information down for my wife. She can look it over when she gets home." Al finished typing as the woman began to speak.

"Oh, I'm sorry." The secretary, caught off guard, did not know how to respond.

"Why are you sorry? It's not your fault she's late." Al ended the phone call by hanging up without further pleasantries.

The next morning at eleven, he and Elaine held a check for $5,000. Al had always paid for everything himself since he was an adolescent. To accept money as a gift, even if it was inherited, was a humbling experience and he was grateful that he only had to speak with the secretary of the law firm.

"This is a new experience for me, but if we were looking for a sign, this would be it. I don't think there is any need to consider putting our home on the market this year." Elaine stared down at the check in disbelief.

"Who would have thought this miracle would have happened. That poor woman was alone in that house and never failed to have a smile on her face and food for breakfast, lunch, and dinner breaks." Al smiled at the memory of his old construction boss and their rapport.

Upon returning home, after depositing the check, Elaine noticed the car previously parked across the street from the house in the same spot. It was a nondescript blue sedan with a white male behind the wheel holding what looked like a camera. He seemed to staring at their house when he wasn't taking pictures.

"Al, it's that car again. Do you think I should call the police?" Elaine stared at the man in the car who looked down into his lap.

"I can go out and talk to him if you want. Maybe he used to stay here when the house was a lodge or he's doing some historical research on places Babe Ruth stayed. He might know me from work and someone told him I got hurt." Al opened the car door and approached the spot Elaine described.

Elaine jumped out of the car. "Al, be careful. That guy doesn't look like he's old enough to have stayed at this house when it was a lodge. I saw him with a camera."

Elaine stood next to the driver's side door and watched Al walk with his cane to the car. Al was halfway around the curve in the driveway, when he heard the car engine start up and the tires on the asphalt roll as the car pulled away.

"Elaine, call the cops," Al called over his shoulder knowing his wife would still be standing next to the car watching him.

An officer was dispatched within fifteen minutes. He walked up to the couple and noticed immediately that Al was blind. "Are you Mr. and Mrs. Plevier?"

Al inclined his head toward the officer. "Yes, my wife called to report a strange car watching us."

The officer held a pocket-sized spiral notebook with a pen attached and prepared to write down the information given to him. "The radio called said a suspicious car was in the area."

Elaine spoke up nervously. "This is the second time I've seen that car parked across the street from our home. My husband tried to approach the car today, and he drove off." Elaine spoke quickly. "We have had so much going on since my husband's accident that he may have been here before, and I didn't notice him."

"Did you get the license plate?" The officer looked down at his pad as a car approached the house on the road and slowed to a stop just beyond the mailbox.

Elaine saw it immediately. "That's the car."

The officer stopped writing, looked up, and started walking toward the street. When he reached the edge of the driveway, he could see a man behind the wheel bent over in concentration.

He stepped up to the driver's side door without the man looking up. "Can I see your license and registration?"

The startled man looked at the officer in surprise. Momentarily stunned because he could not see where the officer had parked the squad car in the driveway, he did not respond.

"I asked for your license and registration. What are you doing parked on this residential street? Are you visiting someone?

(247)

The officer kept one hand at his side, out of the driver's view.

The man regained his composure and reached for his wallet in his back pocket. "I'm working. Here is my Private Investigator's ID with my license and registration."

"What business do you have here?" The officer took the extended paperwork without looking to authenticate it yet.

"I'm not at liberty to discuss the matter." For emphasis, he lifted the camera in his lap for the officer to view.

The officer's tone became loud and stern. "You need to explain yourself now or you can do that back at the station. This is a residential neighborhood, and your presence has already been noted. Exactly what or who are you investigating?"

The man looked straight ahead through the windshield. "I'm investigating fraud."

The officer looked down at the paperwork in his hand while he continued to questioned the driver. "Uh, huh. What fraud?"

"I've been hired to monitor the lifestyle of a litigant involved in a lawsuit." The driver looked solidly at the officer.

A smirk formed at the corners of the officer's mouth. "You mean the blind guy across the street?"

Beads of sweat began to form on the middle-aged bald man's head. "Yes."

"I can verify the fact that he can't see, and I spent two minutes with the guy." The officer did not try to hide his laughter this time. "Look, you can't sit out here watching these people. You're invading their privacy."

"This is a public road. You have no right to stop me." The man was almost comical in his statement.

The officer lost his sense of humor and patience. "You're right, but I can stop you from parking here. Would you like a warning or a ticket?"

The man behind the wheel started the engine. "I'll be happy to move."

"Good. I'll send an extra patrol car down here for the next week or so, to make sure you haven't changed your mind. Have a nice day." The officer stepped back from the car as it drove away, watched until it was back on the adjacent highway, and then walked up the driveway to Al and Elaine.

"What does he want with our house?" Al spoke when he heard the officer approach on the gravel.

"It's not your house he is interested in. It's you, Mr. Plevier. He said he was hired as a private investigator. Are you're involved in a lawsuit?"

Al's face lost all expression. "You're kidding me."

The officer felt sorry for the young couple in front of him who looked shocked, confused, and angry. "No, I'm not. He had a camera on his lap. You've probably been photographed many times. You might want to call your attorney and let him know this is happening. I'm sure it won't be the last time."

Al held up his hands in supplication. "What is the company going to gain by watching me and my family?"

The officer pushed his hat back on his head. "My guess is to see if you're faking it."

"How do you fake being blind?" Al clenched and unclenched his fists.

"I don't know what happened to you folks, but you're obviously involved in a serious legal battle." He looked at the scared faces in front of him. "Do you still want to file a report?" He pulled his notepad from his back pocket.

Elaine switched her puzzled look from Al to the officer. "I don't know. What good would it do?"

"It won't deter whoever hired him, but I don't think he will park in front of your house again. He'll probably be more creative in his approach. If you file a report, you will at least have a record of his plate, and the car will be reported as a suspicious."

"If you think it will do any good, go ahead." Al shifted his weight from one foot to the other and felt like he was acting in a Perry Mason episode.

People watching me, the cops following them, my pregnant wife a nervous wreck as she tries to get the low down from the investigating officer. All this over money?

"What type of lawsuit? What happened?" The officer felt

(249)

comfortable enough with the young couple to ask.

"Industrial accident. Burned and blinded me." Al spoke flatly to the cop as he continued to shift from one foot to the other. "I wonder how long this has been going on? My wife noticed him a day or two ago."

Elaine held her arms over her stomach thinking about the new baby and looked at the officer standing between them and his patrol car. "This is getting scary. What's next? Taps on our phones?"

"That may have already happened, but it's against the law, so I am going to make a suggestion that you have the phone company come out here to check the lines. Have you heard any unusual noises on your line, when you pick up or when a call you're making connects?"

Still holding her arms, she shrugged her shoulders. "I haven't heard anything noticeable or I would have mentioned it to Al." She looked down at her shoes and then at Al, still shifting around where he stood. "I want to make the report. Officer, did you get the agency's name?"

The officer nodded his head yes and then remembered the man in front of him could not see the gesture. "I have everything I need. You can pick up a copy of my report tomorrow."

Al extended his right hand to the officer. "I should walk around the property without my glasses and shirt. If the private detective wants pictures, he can have some good ones."

Elaine saw the officer's expression become sympathetic as he grasped Al's hand and shook it without vigor. "I'll make my captain aware of the situation. Like I said, this is probably not the end, but we can chase the driver away if he parks here."

Elaine turned her head to look across the river behind their house. "I don't know why he bothered sitting in front of the house. You can see perfectly into our home from the other side of the river."

The experienced, middle-aged officer looked at the river and then the young couple. "Maybe the company that hired him didn't think of that, yet."

(250)

Chapter XX: Reminders

*D*aily, Elaine would scan the yard and surrounding areas, looking for the private investigator. It still unnerved her to know that without her knowledge or permission, a stranger was photographing her family in their most private moments. Al fared better with the understanding that it was 'just business'. Fiscally, it did not make sense to him. He spoke to their attorney immediately after filing the report with the police and asked him to contact the defendants in the case. Al proposed that instead of paying the private investigator, the money should be allocated toward a settlement and close the case early. The lawyer lost his patience with Al and explained how he needed his client to deal with the case in a framework of reality, or it would be hard on everyone. The plaintiff, he explained, would never agree to something that ludicrous. Beyond the immediate financial loss at stake for the defendants, was the fact that the company being sued did not want to set a precedent. Al conceded that he understood that common sense was not the vein of a litigious society, and he would acquiesce to his lawyer.

Unlike Elaine, Al didn't give the invasion of his privacy another thought as he moved on. It was another aspect of his new life that he had no control over. On the one-year anniversary of the accident, he sat on the red sofa in the living room learning how to organize his money. The disastrous sale of the Pontiac taught him a valuable lesson, and he took no further chances. Elaine would initially sort the bill denominations for him and he developed a system so he could distinguish them.

This one is a $1 bill because it's folded in half. Here's another $1 and a $5, because it's in half and then folded long ways. I would be lost without Elaine to tell me what I was folding. I got a $20 folded in half twice, and two $10s folded in half and then diagonal. So, I have a total of $47.

He stacked the bills, still folded in their proper order, and placed them back into his wallet. *This isn't much, but it will help me to find some perfume or something for her birthday.* He finished slipping the wallet in his back pocket and heard Elaine approach. "How ya doing, Chubby?"

Approaching her sixth month of pregnancy, Elaine's middle had expanded proportionately. "Fine. I was sorting through old baby clothes. I hope this is a boy because we certainly are prepared."

"Would you like to go out to dinner for your birthday this year?" In a flash of brilliance, Al realized he could avoid shopping.

She smiled brightly and sat down next to him on the couch. "Sure, but aren't you planning ahead a bit? Besides, you still have to make up for forgetting our anniversary." She moved over to make room for Albert, who ran into the room and climbed onto the couch.

Al put his arm around her. "I thought by planning so far ahead for your birthday, all would be forgiven." He kissed her and felt Albert climb behind them.

Elaine reached behind her. "Albert's going to be climbing trees and playing baseball before we know it."

Al felt his stomach twist a little at the thought of not being able to see his active son grow. "He's a bundle of energy, God bless him. Do me a favor."

(252)

"Sure, what?" Albert flopped into Elaine's lap after tumbling over her shoulder.

"After he takes a bath, put my shampoo back in the left corner of the tub, please. Yesterday, I grabbed his toy, and it took an extra ten minutes before I found my stuff." The quick change of subject spirited away thoughts of self-pity.

"Sorry about that. He plays with everything when he's in the tub." Elaine watched Albert climb contentedly into his father's arms.

Al tickled Albert and the little boy squirmed to get away. "You want me to take him outside?" He was still apprehensive about being outside alone with the toddler. "You could come with us and we could push him on the swing."

"Dr. Grove doesn't want you outside without cover." She coaxed Albert to follow his dad.

"I know. I've been doing it a little at a time each day. I can't help it. It feels so good that I'm dreading another damp, cold winter." The smell of decaying leaves and the river met them through the kitchen screen door.

Elaine pretended to chase the little boy who ran immediately toward Al. "How do you feel about today?" She had been avoiding the subject of the date.

Al stood stock still. "I wish I could stay in bed and pull the covers over my head." The minute he awakened this morning, visions of the events from last year replayed themselves. "I feel as though I've aged forty years." Al waited at the back door for her.

Elaine walked past him, as he held the door open for her. She watched their son hurry down the kitchen stairs in the direction of the wooden swing Al had hung for him the first summer he did not have sight. "We'll get through this day."

He followed behind her. "Man, that sun feels good. I never fully appreciated it before."

Elaine picked up Albert and placed him onto the seat. "Al, you worry me." Albert squealed with delight as his Mom pushed him higher and higher.

"I'll go inside in a little while and put on the headphones.

(253)

A couple records should drown out the day for me." Al was grateful the unbearable headaches had ceased, and that he was now able to enjoy the music that gave him solace before the accident.

Elaine wanted to get through today any way possible. "Whatever it takes."

Al stayed outside a little while longer, amazed at how long his son enjoyed being pushed. "I'm going inside. Have fun you two." He counted his steps to the car which was always parked in the same spot, tapped a tire with his cane, and then walked up the steps.

I'll set up five or six albums next to the stereo. I hope Elaine didn't mix them back up after we spent all that time last week organizing them.

He placed his cane in its permanent spot next to the back door, crossed the kitchen, and entered the living room where the entertainment center was. *I need to erase this day. Why did I have to be so good at my job? If I had left earlier, all that would have happened is that I would have been called in, there would've been a mess to clean up, and some guys to fire. Those three guys were on the safe side of the pump and I was on the side that wrecked my life and nearly killed me. Bastards don't even care how my family's doing.*

He eased himself down onto the gold area rug in front of the stereo. He sat recalling the visit he and Elaine had made to the plant a week earlier. He had made her drive him there under the pretense of picking up paperwork with information needed for the lawsuit. In reality, he really wanted to confront the men that had all but forgotten him.

Al and Elaine walked into the front offices and the room went silent. "Hi Girls. Is Mr. Milano around? He was supposed to meet us here with the papers our attorney requested." Elaine had no trouble finding her voice, only controlling her anger.

The older secretary, who had worked for the company over a decade, lifted a file off her desk and brought it to them. She handing it across the high counter that kept visitors out of the office area while she looked away from Elaine. "Here you go."

Elaine took the file as the woman practically let it fall onto the counter. "Thanks."

Al heard the woman's tone and jumped in. "Where's Milano? Out for the day?" He didn't try to contain his sarcasm. "How about Matt? He around anywhere?"

Another secretary still seated, looked up nervously and answered. "It's pretty busy in here. I guess you picked the wrong day to stop by. I'll tell them you were here and picked up the information you requested."

"Wouldn't be the first time I picked the wrong day to come to the plant, now would it?" Al grabbed Elaine's arm and he tapped his cane loudly as he followed her.

Elaine glared over her shoulder. "Thanks for all your help, girls."

Al was not anxious about the visit to A&K, but, as he left the building, he felt a chill run down his spine and the hairs on the back of his neck stood up. "At least I'm leaving through the right door this time."

He pushed so hard on the glass entry door that it swung open ferociously and slammed the brick wall behind it. The secretaries and Elaine took in quick breaths waiting for it to shatter.

When they were in the parking lot next to the car, Elaine breathed out heavily. "Al, we shouldn't have come here. I should have told you no. The papers could have been mailed."

He shook his head. "I needed to come here one last time." I'm not sure what I was expecting." He heard the familiar click of the door opening, grabbed at the handle, and almost hit Elaine. "Maybe part of me hoped that someone would show some concern for my family." He slipped into the familiar seat. "Those people act like the struggles we have faced the last year are not important to anyone outside our family."

"Easy. We're getting out of here." She walked around the front of the car and caught movement in a window that faced the parking lot. The figure of a man who had been standing and watching them slid into the shadows of the room's interior. *It's a year later and that man is still hiding.* She walked around the car and slipped behind the wheel. "Al, we're together."

"Let's get out of here. I almost gave my life to this place."

Al shook his head in anger and let his memories retreat as he returned to the present. He grabbed two albums. During the summer evenings that he and Elaine spent organizing their extensive album collection, he had used the Braille system to mark each album jacket. He had placed the tape with the titles on the upper right corner. Lying on the carpet and trying to block out the day he expected to be blasted into another world.

I'd better make sure the headphones are plugged in.

He followed the cord that was firmly connected on the face of the stereo, placed a record on the turntable, put the phones on his head, and turned the volume knob all the way to the right. The music kicked on and blared out so loud that he was sure the world would melt away today. Unfortunately, it was one of Elaine's and its sentimental message blasted too loud to be taken seriously.

He was laughing hysterically with the headphones blaring as she stood over him. *I'll pretend I never saw him.*

"Daddy!" Albert wriggled out of her arms, ran over, and pulled at the 'big ears' his Dad was wearing.

Al sat up straight, pushed the headphones completely off and then heard his giggling son. "Hey, you." He gained control of himself and knew that if he had eye ducts to shed tears, tears of laughter would have been running down his face.

Elaine could hear the music blaring from the headphones. "Why are you listening to my music?"

Al shook his head still laughing. "I grabbed the wrong one." Albert giddily rolled off his dad and began to run circles around him. "It's over Elaine."

Relieved that he had moved past the day she joined him on the floor. "This day was going to be rough no matter what."

"No. I mean the whole mess. It knocked us down and regurgitated our lives, but it didn't beat us."

He breathed out heavily. "I'm still laughing."

She smirked agreeably. "If anyone has a right to laugh at their lives and keep going, it's us."

Chapter XXI: Gifts

*T*ime continued its old habit of passing quickly for the young family as the holidays drew near for the second time in their new life. Routine and familiarity replaced the drama of the previous year, allowing Al the comfort of progressing in all areas of living without sight. The only challenge he was unable to conquer before the holidays was Braille reading. Lee Peterson worked with him using every technique at his disposal and although he considered Al a quick study, he told him he was the worst Braille student he had ever had. Al ended up destroying the books by picking the raised dots off the page with his insensitive fingers. By the end of their sessions, he and Lee had become good friends and spent more time together hanging out talking about sports than practicing his life skills.

Thanksgiving, Christmas, and Elaine's birthday stood starkly in front of them. On November 26, at six in the evening, as Elaine and Al discussed the holiday dinner to be held at Elaine's parents, there was a knock on the front door. Fenna's mother-in-law and father in law stood before Elaine with a fully cooked Thanksgiving dinner for ten.

"We didn't want you to consider cooking and thought you might like to invite Elaine's family over." The couple pushed past

(257)

a stunned and teary-eyed Elaine.

"Your Mom can heat this stuff up without having to cook it. The entire meal is wrapped and ready for the table. We'll put it in the fridge for you." The smiling woman went moved about with precision.

Al struggled for words and felt humility wash over him for the second time that year. "You are wonderful. Thank you so much."

Fenna's mother-in-law spoke first. "This is our gift to you. Enjoy it. We'll be at Fenna's letting her cook for us, and trying to get some quality time with their kids."

Elaine made a pot of coffee and talked with the couple until it was time for Albert to be put to bed. Everyone hugged, wished each other Happy Thanksgiving as a sense of the inability to ever repay such a kindness enveloped both Al and Elaine. Al felt his spirits lift as the smell of tomorrow's meal assaulted his senses.

"We are blessed." He then turned to the fridge to steal stuffing.

Elaine smiled as she watched him hanging onto the fridge door. "I saw the stress that has been on your face dissolve into laughter. I know the holidays don't hold the same excitement for you that they used to, but now we can stay home, relax and enjoy a home-cooked meal." Elaine laughed at his stuffed cheeks. "Oh, I'd better call Mom to let her know."

"I have a feeling Bob already told them. Bob's parents wouldn't let your mom buy and prepare all that food ahead of time." Al left the fridge door open as he turned to get a plate and a fork. "The surprise was for us."

"Save some for tomorrow and for me." Elaine walked quickly to get her own fork. The two of them jockeyed for a spot while each stabbed at tomorrow's dinner.

Mrs. Hinds did know about Elaine's surprise and the next day brought over pies she had cooked. The family was able to relax and even ate and drink with disposable dinnerware. It was a true dinner of gratitude that set a tone for the rest of the holiday season.

On Christmas Eve Elaine, three weeks before her due date, Elaine watched Albert tear through gift paper at her parent's home.

Mrs. Hinds held out a small plate with hors-d'oeuvres. "Elaine, eat."

Elaine took the bright red plastic plate full of food her mother offered her and indicated with her chin where Al sat on the gold carpet with Albert. "Look at my two men. It's hard to believe we'll have another little one this time next year." She took a bite of the cracker with cheese.

Mrs. Hinds looked at Al, who sat on the carpet trying in vain to keep Albert's attention on one toy at a time. "That child is not going to stop bouncing off the walls until he falls asleep under the tree tomorrow night."

Elaine rested her plate on her stomach. "It's going to be a long toy ride for the next decade."

Mrs. Hinds studied Elaine's glowing face. "What is the doctor's latest prognosis for the corneal transplant? Have you two gotten some good news?"

Elaine smiled broadly. "We still have to get through the plastic surgery in January for his chest reconstruction. The doctor was waiting to perform that surgery until Al had regained his strength and weight, and was past the cause of the severe headaches. When Al has a clean bill of health, we can begin to work toward getting on the transplant list. We have a few hurdles, but it is possible." Elaine looked over at Al playing with Albert. "Mom, Al can see fractured light during his visits to the optometrist. That is a very good indication that the corneal transplant will be a success."

"I'm so happy for you both." The two women embraced and Elaine felt that her family was moving forward, no matter how slow the pace would be.

That night Al carried a sleeping Albert into the house and then set the presents under the tree before going to bed. Albert woke before his parents on Christmas morning and immediately ran to the tree. His squeals, the sound of paper being torn, and boxes tossed, catapulted both of them out of bed.

scrambling for the camera. Little Albert's joy and energy kept him the focus of the day. Unbeknownst to him, it would be the last Christmas he didn't have to share his parents with another sibling as he blissfully played into a state of exhaustion. His sleeping form was lifted out from underneath the tree by mid-afternoon.

Elaine and Al sat together for a respite in front of the tree with Al's one hand on Elaine's stomach and the other behind his head. "We can do this."

"Merry Christmas, Al."

"Merry Christmas, Sweetheart." He leaned his head back comfortably without the headaches of the previous year. "Now we can start concentrating on the arrival of the new baby."

Al began to mark the days before the birth of the new baby on his calendar with Braille. By January 21, he was nervous. "Elaine, we need to have a game plan in case the baby comes in the middle of the night. Is your mom ready to be on call?'

"Yes, but I already know the day I need her." She folded the laundry Al had brought up for her.

"A-a-r-r you in labor now?" He stood still.

She rolled her eyes and carried a small pile of Albert's clothes toward the hall. "Do you think I would be this relaxed if I was in labor? My doctor called. He wants to start his vacation on the twenty-third so he's going to induce tomorrow if I don't go into labor on my own."

"Nice guy." Al sat back and breathed out.

"The minute you came into the kitchen." She rubbed her lower back. "At least we can plan ahead. My mom is going to drive us and Dad will stay here with Albert in the morning. Your mom or your sister will take over in the afternoon." She looked down at her stomach. "I'm ready to have this baby."

Al smiled at Elaine. "I'm really getting excited. We have to get you packed."

"My suitcase is packed and dinner is my last full meal if I am going to be induced first thing in the morning." She carried another small armful of clothes into their bedroom.

"What will it be? I'll cook." He smiled broadly at her.

(260)

She stifled her laughter. "How about pizza?"

"Perfect." Al reached for the phone. "When are your parents getting here tomorrow?"

"Around seven o'clock. We want to get to the hospital and check in by eight."

Al smiled over at her. "Good. Having your mom with me will make the time pass quicker. When Albert was born, I felt like I was never going to leave the waiting room."

Elaine shot him an incredulous look she was glad he could not see. "Sorry to make you wait. Time passed so quickly for me."

Al winced. "Ooh, sorry."

The next morning, Al and his mother-in-law were seated in the maternity ward waiting room. "Mom, thank you for all you do for us. It makes life easy and more enjoyable."

"Al, family does for family. Think about everything that you've done for us. Remember the roof? You seriously don't think your father-in-law could have fixed that for us in the rain. What about when he was sick? You took a day off from work to visit him in the hospital."

"You guys have been great to me since the first day Elaine brought me home to meet you." He whistled lowly. "Man, was I nervous. I never thought I was good enough for Elaine."

"We did." Mrs. Hinds stoically went back to the magazine she was leafing through.

A nurse came into the waiting room. "Mr. Plevier?"

"Yes?" Al jumped out of his seat.

"You can go in now. Your wife is doing fine." The young woman knew a little about the family history and found tears forming in her eyes.

"What do we have?" Al started to shift from foot to foot.

"I'll let her tell you about the newest member of your family. The baby is in the room with her." The nurse took his hand and put it through her arm. "I'll take you in."

"Mom, do you mind waiting?" Al felt guilty leaving Elaine's mother behind.

Mrs. Hinds had gotten up to stand next to Al, but sat back

down. "Al, this is your time, enjoy it."

The nurse started to lead Al and he stopped her short. "Wait, I need my cane."

He was led down the hall to Elaine. "Hi Al," came a tired voice.

"Hi." Al could hardly speak as he walked toward Elaine's voice and stood next to the bedside.

The nurse was looking for the opportunity to excuse herself. "Mr. Plevier, the bassinet is on the other side of the bed. Elaine can direct you. I'll leave you two alone."

Al waited to hear the padded shoes leave the room. "How are you?" She met him halfway for a kiss as he leaned toward her.

"I'm fine. Meet your new son." Elaine felt the warm comfort of her own family unit.

Al tried to hide the constriction of his throat. "Another boy. We are so blessed. I can't believe it." He felt his way around the hospital bed very carefully.

"He is next to the right side of my bed about three feet from the end." She stared at her new baby peacefully bundled.

Al ran his hand around the bed as he walked. "Am I close?"

"Yes. Put your hands out." Elaine watched Al move toward the baby with the pride a new mother feels.

Al felt the side of a hospital bassinet. "There you are."

"Al, he's perfect. Ten fingers, ten toes. He has big blue eyes that are drinking in the world." With her blond hair still matted to her forehead, Elaine had the glow of having given birth.

Al heard a small sound coming from the bassinet. "What's he doing?"

"I think he may be getting ready for his first feeding." She adjusted herself in the bed to watch the baby more closely.

A nurse came into the recovery room. "We're going to move you to your room now, Mrs. Plevier. You can come too, Dad. Congratulations."

Al used his finger and traced an outline of the baby's face. "Thank you. His name is Lawrence." He tried to step back out of the way as he heard movement in the room.

The nurse came close and placed a hand gently on Al's shoulder. "You're fine. I'm going to take the little guy to the nursery and get him settled in. Mr. Plevier, please follow close behind. We'll keep an eye on you."

Elaine grabbed Al's hand as the bed rolled past him. "I can't believe we have two boys."

Al felt his throat constrict. "I love you guys. I can't wait until Albert sees his little brother." He wondered how the active two-year-old would feel about sharing his parents' attention. "I should go get your mother."

One of the male orderlies saw Al's need for assistance. "If you follow us into the room, after I get your wife settled I'll take you down to the waiting room."

He kept his hand on the shoulder of the orderly as Elaine's bed was pushed into her new room. When she was settled in Al kissed her goodbye and the younger of the two orderlies made conversation as he guided Al back to the waiting area. "What happened? Nam?"

"Huh?" The young man caught Al off guard. "Oh, you mean my eyes?"

"I saw the burns on your hands too." The young man didn't stop to consider what he said. His eyes were wide with the anticipation of a guts and glory scene.

Oh, this guy is special. "Nothing that sensational. Job related. Boring, really."

"That sucks." The two finished the short walk in silence.

"Make a left here. I'll hold the door for you. The waiting room is straight ahead. Your mother-in-law will see you as soon as the door opens."

"Thanks. Do you have the time to tell my mother-in-law the way back? I was trying to count my steps and the turns we made, but I'm so excited about the baby that I got distracted." Al heard the door open and felt the young man step to the side.

"I'll walk you both back. There's probably nothing for me to do." The young man sounded bored.

(263)

"Thanks." He moved past the orderly and his mother-in-law looked up.

She walked toward a smiling Al. "Do I have a granddaughter or grandson?"

"You have another handsome grandson." He reached out and gave her a quick hug. "Elaine is fine and she tells me the baby is perfect. Let's go see them."

The young man walked them back to Elaine's room. "Good luck, man. Have fun with the kid."

"Thanks." *Hope I never run into that guy in an alley.*

Mrs. Hinds walked over to her daughter. "Hi, Honey. How are you?"

"Tired and uncomfortable. You have to go see the baby. Lawrence is perfect." Elaine closed her eyes.

"I'll take Al down to the nursery with me. You rest. We'll see you later. We have a lot of calls to make." She turned to put her arm through Al's.

"And flowers to buy. You have to get me to the gift shop." He felt like a little kid on his birthday.

Al and his mother-in-law spent several long minutes at the nursery window with Mrs. Hinds describing every tiny movement the new baby made. "Al, his eyes are wide open."

"I can't wait to hold him. I was so nervous with Albert." He shifted his weight continuously from one foot to the other.

"You've had plenty of practice since then." The older woman continued to stare through the glass at the baby. "Elaine is lucky to have you home to help."

"I guess that means I can't get out of changing diapers this time." They were quiet. "I'll see him, Mom, don't worry. Once I have my corneal transplant, I'll see them both."

A nurse came to the window and motioned for Mrs. Hinds to show her which baby she and Al were there to see. Mrs. Hinds pointed to Lawrence and then the nurse motioned for them to come to the nursery entrance. "Mr. Plevier?"

"Yes?" Al couldn't imagine what the nurse wanted.

The nurse smiled understandingly. "I wanted to know if

you would like to come inside and hold him. We never allow it, but I thought you might want some special pointers." The nurse was a professional and believed she was instructing the new father with the disability, not as a favor, but as part of her job.

"Thank you." Al didn't care what her reasons were. He just wanted to hold his son.

The nurse turned to Mrs. Hinds. "I'm sorry. You'll have to wait here." The nurse brought Al into the first room and gave him a mask and gown to slip over his clothes. "You can wash your hands over here." She led Al to a sink with antiseptic soap and waited until he finished. "Now, come with me."

Al was enveloped with the scent of a baby as soon as he entered the bassinet area. He heard soft baby noises and also a couple of screamers toward the back of the room. The nurse led him to a rocker and asked him to sit down and assume the cradling position. Before long, he felt a small bundle placed in his arms.

"Hello, Lawrence." Joy ran through his veins as the baby made a kitten sound.

"He's bundled nice and tight." The nurse stood watching the young father.

Al felt the weight of the bundle as he held him close. "I'm your dad."

I feel the joy. He is perfect. I never appreciated the weight of Albert in my arms. This little guy has substance. I can feel his strength. Al took his index finger and touched the baby's clenched fist sticking through the top of the blanket and he grasped it in response. *He is strong.*

"By next year you and your brother are going to be tearing the house apart." A lump started to form in his throat."

"Mr. Plevier, would you like to feed him?"

Al wondered if Elaine would like to be the first to feed him and then decided to go for it. "Yes, I would love to."

The nurse moved the bottle into his right hand and eased the nipple toward the baby's mouth.

"You're doing fine. Very good for your first baby." The nurse misunderstood Al's shyness.

(265)

"This is actually our second. I lost my sight after our first son was born." He could hear the baby sucking down the bottle. "Boy, this guy is hungry." He felt the infant stop sucking. The baby spit out the nipple and let out the first cry his father heard. "That's a strong set of lungs you have. Your mom and I will take good care of you. Thank you for being born. Welcome to the world, Lawrence. We're really glad you're here."

Chapter XXII: Children

$\mathscr{L}$awrence was brought home three days later, welcomed with joy, and instantly referred to as Larry. Al's next surgery to reconstruct the right side of his chest cavity was scheduled for three weeks after Larry's birth, and he was overwhelmed with guilt knowing that his wife would have a newborn, a toddler, and a recovering husband to care for. He could do nothing to avoid the burden.

The day of the surgery, Al waited for Elaine's mother and sister to arrive. "Elaine, I know we'll have lots of help when I come home, but I don't want you to think I'll be lying on the couch. I will be in the hospital for a week, so that should give my body plenty of time to get over the initial pain and immobility." He held Larry while sitting on the floor as Albert played around them. "You're still recovering from Larry's birth, and I don't want you overdoing it."

Elaine sipped the juice she had left from breakfast. "I'm fine. I've recovered beautifully these last three weeks. With both boys, I couldn't have made the transition without you. I don't' know what I'm going to do while you're in the hospital."

Al snuggled Larry. "I hate the idea of leaving the three of you." Albert climbed onto the couch and leaned over Al's shoulder. "Watch out for the baby, big guy." He let Albert wrap his arms around his neck while he continued the conversation with Elaine. "If you are ever too tired to come during visiting hours, I understand. Don't exhaust yourself with driving. Initially, I'll be out of it from the pain medication."

"This is the first time you aren't being admitted under an emergency basis." Elaine admired how accepting Al was each time he had to be readmitted for a procedure.

"I consider this a stop gap to getting my sight back. I want that more than anything. I can't wait to look at you and the kids." Al felt Albert trying to get his dad to wrestle with him.

"Albert, come on over here while Daddy holds Larry." Elaine wrapped an arm around Albert's waist to try and contain him. Immediately, he grabbed his father harder and started to scream. She smiled and instead of corralling him, decided to take Larry from Al. "I'll see if I can get Larry to take part of a bottle."

Al pulled Albert onto his lap. The little boy burst into giggles and squirmed to climb behind him. "I think the biggest challenge is going to be getting Albert to understand that Daddy won't be able to play for a while." Al ran his free hand through his hair. It already had begun to feel oily since his shower this morning. "I swear my hair is thinner now. Tell me the truth, am I going bald?"

She laughed from the kitchen. "No." As she reached for her tea, the back door opened. "Hi, Mom."

Mrs. Hinds stepped into the doorway with Ronnie behind her. "Hi. You two ready to go?"

"Almost. I'm putting a bottle on for Larry. I thought it would satisfy him and make it easier for you as we leave."

Ronnie dropped her purse onto the kitchen counter. "That kid isn't even going to notice you're gone."

Elaine held her tongue and looked over at her mom. "Mom

would you please take the baby when we leave? Ronnie can keep Albert occupied."

"Still giving out orders." Ronnie shot over her shoulder as she walked into the living room where Albert still played with his dad. "Come on, Cutie. Let me see those new pictures mommy said you drew on your bedroom walls. Maybe we can make some pictures of our own." She smiled, picked up Albert and tickled him.

Elaine rolled her eyes as she kneeled down on the carpet with Al and Larry. "She's the cool aunt."

"No doubt." Al eased the baby to Elaine in a handoff as he felt her arms gather around the bundle.

Mrs. Hinds walked over and smiled down at the new baby. "Ronnie is giving you a hard time, but she was looking forward to spending time with the boys." She handed a new bottle to Elaine.

Larry needed no encouragement as Elaine placed the bottle to his lips. "He's going to be a bruiser." She smiled lovingly at the baby.

Al walked into the kitchen where his hospital suitcase sat. "We should get going now that your mom is here. Is it still snowing?"

Elaine gently handed Larry off to her mom and he cried immediately. "The snow is starting to come down a little heavier. Be careful. The roads are covered." Mrs. Hinds struggled to be heard over the annoyed baby. "Al, good luck. We're praying for you, as always."

"Thanks, Mom. It's probably better if we sneak out of here without Albert seeing us go." Al was already slipping on his coat.

Elaine kissed the baby on the forehead. "Thanks, Mom. I'll call you in a couple of hours."

Due to snow conditions, the forty-five-minute drive to Hackensack Hospital took three hours. Elaine did not bother to stop at a phone booth on the way, assuming the hospital personnel would realize the reason for their delay.

Al, on the other hand, felt his anxiety the longer the car ride grew. "I hate this surgery, but at least I'm not at Overlook. Even the smell of that place gives me nightmares."

"I understand. It should only be another fifteen minutes. We're crawling along, but I can see the hospital."

Elaine thought it would take a half hour to bring him upstairs. She was caught unprepared to say goodbye when the desk nurse called for an orderly with a wheelchair.

Al quickly tried to squeeze in a goodbye. "Sorry for the long drive, Hon. I love you." She leaned into him for a kiss as the orderly came with the wheelchair.

Al kissed her back. "Me too."

The heavy-set orderly with a friendly face tried to coax them along. "Your entourage is waiting upstairs for you."

"We planned on being here two hours ago, but the snow slowed us down." The morning's misadventure played out in his mind.

"Bye, Al." Elaine was still surprised at how she felt cold fear whenever she had to leave him for surgery.

"Bye, Sweetheart. See you soon." Al was no longer afraid of anything.

The orderly started to pull him away.

"Hold up a minute." Al dropped a foot onto the floor from the footrests to stop the chair.

"What's wrong, Mr. Plevier?" The orderly thought the man was in pain.

Al hesitated and gripped the arms of the wheelchair. "Look, I've been in and out of hospitals for the last year and a half, and it's always the same. Without sight, I'm at a disadvantage. If my wife isn't next to me wherever I'm being taken, I lose my sense of security. If you have to dump me with someone else, I need to know where we are, the time, and who I am being passed off to."

The good-natured professional began to push the chair. "Sure. You'll be with me today until your prep begins." The reassurance the orderly offered was authentic and compassionate.

"Good, thanks." Al relaxed into the chair seat.

(270)

"I'm Michael." The man smiled down at Al's head.

"Let's roll, Michael." His apprehension over the procedure began to dissipate.

Al was wheeled upstairs to the operating room and sedated within the hour. While under anesthesia, his dreams took him back to Paterson, NJ where he was born. In the dream, he was a child of twelve running with his group of pals. The boys were jumping from rooftop to rooftop of the apartment buildings where each member of the group lived. The narrow alleys offered only enough space for one person to walk through on the street level and wide enough at the roof to entertain the daring escapades of preteen boys. A recent snowfall added to the thrill and didn't slow the group down. It was close to supper time, and Al knew his grandmother would be looking for him if he didn't show up on time.

"Come on you guys. That old lady will chase me with the broom if I'm late." His feet hit the roof of the building next to his and the chimney smoke burned his eyes.

"You got time. We're almost to your building." His best friend, Frankie, was right on Al's heels.

"Let's get there quick," Al yelled over his shoulder. "We can hang out behind my chimney and throw snowballs at the people on the street." He closed his eyes tight against the smoke and opened them when he knew he was halfway across the roof.

A chorus of the five boy's voices answered from the edge of the other building. "People on the street will never see us!"

Frankie continued his banter with Al. "Hey, Plev? Your grandma is one tough broad for a short lady. Do ya think she'll ever lose that accent? What is that anyway?"

"Italian. Right off the boat." He picked up speed and leaped across the expanse between the rooftops. He felt like Superman.

"I thought you were Dutch? You said that in school. You Lyin' to Mr. Boneyard?" Frankie landed next to him in seconds.

"You're an idiot, Frankie. Grandma Padula's my mom's old lady. My dad's parents are dead, but they were Dutch." Al ran

(271)

to get ahead of the others, so he could claim the best drift of snow for cover. He knew where it was from experience, and he headed directly behind the chimney, five feet away.

Frankie's limited view of the world divided all ethnicities by their corresponding Paterson neighborhoods. "Man, half of ya lives in Stony Road section and the other half lives in…" Frankie never got to finish his sentence.

"I should kick your butt." Al formed a snowball the size of a baseball.

"Plev, you got the best angle up here for cars." Frankie snuck next to Al and started to scoop snow.

He gave his friend the death look, and Frankie backed away from his spot. Al's defenses were up, and he had to prove himself better than his friends. "I have more fun than you guys. Only person watchin' me right after school is the old lady, and she's so busy with the laundry and house stuff that I sneak out all the time. I just have to be on time for supper." He wiped his nose with the back of his shirt sleeve. He bent quickly to his pile and thought he pulled a muscle in his right arm. "Ouch."

Frankie gave Al a know it all look. "But when she's mad, you better run. I saw her get so mad at you one time, I thought that gold tooth would come poppin' right outta her mouth. All four feet of her was jumpin' up and down lookin' like she was spittin' while she talked." Frankie laughed as he worked hard on his pile never noticing that his slicked-back hair was sticking to his head.

Al laughed with Frankie and felt like he was free. "She's afraid I'm gonna end up a hood 'cause we got no money and my dad is dead." The rest of the boys had reached Al's roof and started to create a stockpile of ammunition. "When I get old, I'm gonna have a house and it's gonna have lots of bedrooms. Sleeping on the couch stinks." He hid behind the roof's half wall and tried to warm up his gloveless hands by breathing on them.

Charlie piped in as he continued to make snowballs. "At least we all got places to stay. Mickey got sent to a home for boys when his mom left and he don't even know where she is." Charlie looked from Al's stockpile to Frankie's and grew jealous. "You're

(272)

fast."

Al moved protectively in front of his pile. "My dad's mom and dad met at an orphanage. I never met them. Died before my dad died." Al went back to work to keep his pile the biggest. He started to laugh uncontrollably. "I used to fill pots up with water and dump them on the people on the street. I'd duck and I could hear them cursin' and swearin' all the way down to Brighton Ave." He stopped laughing. "I got caught once. My grandma beat my butt red." All six boys laughed and then began to throw snowballs off the roof.

"Betcha cried." Charlie had to have the last dig on Al.

"Nope. Somebody woulda found out and then everybody at '7' woulda laughed." Al thought how unlucky it was to have your public school named PS7 and then took aim. "I nailed the Woody! That's what he gets for drivin' that ugly station wagon."

Frankie watched with envy. "You comin' to Great Eastern tomorrow after school?" He smiled at the thought of the local box store that had an arcade section where the kids hung out.

"Yup. I'll be there." Al smirked to himself. My grandma said not to ride my bike or I'll catch it good from her, so I'm pushing my bike and I'll ride it back. It ain't lyin'." Al looked sideways at his friend like a tough guy who outsmarted everybody. "Yesterday she tol' me she didn't want to see me hitchhiking in the street either, so when I hitchhike to da mall, I stand on the sidewalk! That ain't
lyin' neither."

Somewhere in the early evening dusk, he heard his grandma call his name. He knew he must be late for supper, but for some reason, she didn't sound mad, just persistent. Over and over, she called his name until he didn't recognize the voice as hers. Suddenly, the world went black. He was in pain and could not see.

"Albert, it's time to wake up. Wake up. Come on, Albert. You need to wake up now." The gentle recovery nurse kept her voice low and steady.

"I'm awake. Knock me back out." His right side felt like

(273)

it was on fire.

"Dr. Grove said the surgery went very well. Your movement should return to what you had prior to the accident. The intended muscles were pulled from the back to the front. You are stitched in a 'U' shape under your right arm and you should heal in a week or two." The nurse busied herself with the tasks she needed to complete. "The discomfort you are in is perfectly normal."

"Where's my wife?"

"She'll be waiting for you in your room. You're still in recovery." The nurse took his blood pressure. "I have to leave the room. Try to stay awake. If you drift off, I'll wake you."

Al remembered his dream and started to think about his old neighborhood and his childhood friends. *Man, that was some group I used to run with. Hell, we looked out for each other and had good, clean fun. Didn't want to hurt anybody permanently. Everybody took care of everybody. The guys even looked out for Paulie, the retarded kid in my building. We never left out any of the handicapped kids on the block. Never let anybody from another neighborhood bother them either. We had fun. We never got caught 'cause we never did anything bad enough to worry about it. How the hell we ever survived the daily schoolyard fights I'll never know. Beatin' each other up over nothin' in particular.*

The nurse came back. "Albert? Are you with me?"

"Haven't left." He was still very groggy and his voice expressed it. "When am I being moved?"

"In an hour." She checked his tubes and machines monitoring his vitals. "I hear you have a new baby at home."

Al smiled weakly. "He's a real powerhouse. I can tell by his grip."

The middle-aged brunette looked away from Al. "I can still remember holding each of my three boys for the first time. My youngest is in college now."

"Times goes by so quickly." Al started to drift off.

His thoughts returned to his childhood dream. *The boys looked so real. I swear I felt the snow. It was white but with that gray tint from the city. I smelled the smoke from the chimney. Nobody cared if you were poor in that neighborhood, except for that one time and I don't think that kid understood.*

Out of nowhere, the sad memory from an invitation to a childhood birthday party came back to him. But it wasn't the birthday boy that had upset him, it was that big kid from the other street. *Maybe he thought my mom didn't care. I must have been eight or nine. I was a real independent little thing. Mom had to pinch pennies to get that present for the birthday boy. Nice gift too, a Superman lunchbox. I saw that kid bring that to school for two years. He wasn't rich either, but he wasn't poor like we were. I had those hand-me-down clothes that my mom always had to hem. My pants must have looked pretty bad cause that big kid looked me up and down and told me I should have dressed up for the party. He didn't know those were the best clothes I had. I put the present on the table and left. My mom never knew. Man, I hid around every corner I could find until two hours had passed.* Al felt the acute childhood pain. *The world can be cruel if you take it to heart. I don't know what would have become of me without baseball.* He automatically switched to the subject that always carried him through hard times. *"Westside Warriors, my first baseball team. Now that tryout was cold. No glove, no hat, just get up and if you get on base, you're on the team. I made it.*

"Albert, how are you? Still awake?" The same nurse moved to the head of his bed and began to unplug things. "It's time to move." She took his blood pressure one more time and then removed the cuff. Al heard two more people enter the room. "He goes down to 345. His wife will be waiting for him."

The bed began to move slowly. *I feel sick. It must be the anesthesia. I thought I was over this. The elevator might be more than I can handle today.*

"How close are we? Do we have to go in the elevator?"

"A couple more turns." A deep voice responded to him.

The bed slowed down and made a sharp turn. "Hi, Al. How are you?"

"Elaine, I'm sore, as hell. Feel like I been sliced and diced." The two orderlies gently pushed the bed in place.

(275)

The nurse came in to check the progress. "How are we doing folks? Mr. Plevier, are you awake?"

"Wide awake. What time is it?"

Elaine came to the side of the bed. "It's about seven pm." She saw the IV in Al's left arm and didn't take his hand.

He remembered the dreams of this afternoon. "Elaine, I had the best dream. I was twelve back in Paterson with the gang."

She laughed softly. "What were you doing, walking along the tracks or through bum row?"

"We were jumping from roof to roof and throwing snowballs at cars. I could see their faces as if all the boys were standing right in front of me. Grandma was still alive." A wave of sentimentality washed over him as he thought about the pint-sized lady with the mean temper.

Elaine smoothed a few strands of Al's usually close-cropped hair from around his ear. "Must have been the storm we drove through today."

"I wonder whatever happened to those guys?" Al's voice trailed off. "We all divided into other groups by senior year of high school. You took up a lot of my time, and by college, we were all over the place. I heard Frankie went into the service. I hope he made it out of Nam."

I'll ask Mom about those guys. Nah, she won't even remember them. She was always working and my sister was running with her crowd by then. My grandmother would've remembered every one of their faces. She hated my friends and thought I was turning into trouble. She was one tough old lady.

He released himself to the last of the anesthesia and returned to his dream of Paterson. He was free, young, and poor, without a care in the world.

Chapter XXIII: Overdone

The rain had been continuous for three days during Al's first week home after the latest surgery that corrected his chest cavity. The Ramapo River, which ran seventy feet from the back of the house and normally twenty feet below the embankment, had crested. Al and Elaine usually enjoyed the beauty of the river knowing Albert and Larry would be safe behind the fully fenced and gated yard.

Al reached for the back scratcher that was never far from his hand since he arrived home. "When can I wear my Jobe shirt? I can't take much more of this. Ouch!" He reached too far and felt the strain on his incision through the sling.

Elaine handed Albert some toast with one hand and held Larry in the other. "Try to relax. We're all stuck in the house. You'll be able to wear it next week but, in the meantime try not to do further damage to yourself."

Al still felt guilty knowing the workload she had undertaken with an infant, a toddler, and a recovering husband. "Sorry." His thoughts turned to the recent series of heavy rain storms. "Did you check the basement to see if we're getting any water?"

Elaine looked out at the falling rain. "No. I'll ask Dad to stop by after work. I'm sure we have some water. Everything is saturated."

She looked up at the ten-foot, rugged beam ceiling to see a lantern light swinging slightly in the breeze from the open French door. "I'm glad we don't have any leaks."

"What about the fireplace? Anything coming in?" Al knew the potential for leakage around the closed damper.

The living room fireplace had served as the focal point for guests of the former lodge. It was fieldstone from floor to ceiling, had an opening in the hearth fifty-four inches wide and three and a half feet high. The mantel was eight feet across, five and a half feet off the floor and eighteen inches wide.

Elaine glanced over at the hearth. "A little. The rain was a steady driving force this morning."

Al fidgeted. *I need to move around. I'll go down to the basement myself and check."*

"Please be careful. For crying out loud, you just got out of the hospital and your arm is still in a sling. If you slip on the stairs, you could hurt yourself and have to start over." Larry cooed in her arms lessening the exasperation she felt.

He opened the back door without responding and let the rain and cool air play onto his skin. *I'd better take my time.*

The stairs to the basement were enclosed on all sides by cement blocks that matched the foundation of the house. The top of the stairwell was about twenty feet from the kitchen door and was covered by an overhang. Al stepped down from the kitchen stairs and felt his way along the side of the house with his left hand, as the rain showered lightly over him. His right foot found the basement steps and he proceeded downward, one step at a time, keeping his left hand on the wall until he reached the last step and a sensation came over him.

I feel something strange, like a vibration in the air.

He opened the door and started to step down the eight-inch rise of the final step into the basement area. His sneaker touched the water that had gathered there, and he felt an electrical shock.

Jumping up automatically, he landed on top of the washing machine adjacent on the right to the stair he had been standing on and felt pain rip through him as his arm automatically came out of the sling to pull him out of harm's way. Without hesitation, he instinctively pushed himself off the washer, throwing his body through the open doorway and landing flat just outside the door.

"Shit!" Pain from his torn incision overwhelmed him. He half walked, half dragged himself wincing at every movement, up the stairs, to the back steps, and into the kitchen.

Al didn't hear movement in the kitchen. "Elaine?"

"That was fast." Albert stared over his mother's shoulder as she closed the refrigerator door and turned to Al. "Oh, my God, you're bleeding! Why did you pull your arm out of the sling?"

He limped onto a stool and leaned heavily on the counter. "I guess checking on the basement wasn't such a good idea."

"What happened? Never mind. I'll call Sue to watch the boys. We need to get you to the hospital." Elaine's next call was to Dr. Grove who, after listening to her story, lost his temper, and swore loud enough for Al to hear him.

He waited for Elaine to hang up. "He sounds pissed."

Elaine turned to Al and shook her head in disbelief. "Did you try to lift something or did you fall?" She lifted Albert up when he started to whine in response to the commotion.

Al hung his head as he held a dishtowel he grabbed off its regular place on the counter on his wounded body. "I twisted my body when I felt the shock."

"The shock? You were electrocuted?" She stared at him as Albert looked from her to his miserable father.

"No, just shocked. There must be six inches of water throughout the basement. It couldn't have puddled or I wouldn't have felt the current. I jumped up to avoid the water, tore my stitches, and landed face first on the landing." Al's attempt at sympathy did not go far.

Elaine was scared and mad. "I hope you don't have to be operated on again."

He felt the dish towel moisten under his hand. "How bad

(279)

is the blood?"

She walked over and made an assessment. "You're not bleeding profusely, but it's obvious you ripped some of your stitches. Dr. Grove is furious. I never heard him lose his composure before, but I think you're going to get the full brunt of his anger."

Al hung his head a little more. "Great."

The neighbor Elaine had called, breathlessly burst through the back door to find Al still leaning against the counter. "Get to the hospital. The boys will be fine. When was Larry's last bottle?"

"Fifteen minutes ago. He's lying in the playpen, but I'm sure he'll be looking for attention soon." She placed Albert on his feet, shoved her arms into her coat and tried to calm the toddler. "Albert, you have fun with Sue. Mommy and daddy will be back in a little while." She picked up her purse and wrapped Al's coat gently over his shoulders. "Come on, Al."

Elaine and Al arrived at the emergency room of Wayne General Hospital and were admitted immediately. The emergency room on-call doctor could not believe their story as he looked at the destroyed work the plastic surgeon would need to repair. "Of all the stupid things I have ever heard." The staff kept Al comfortable and controlled the bleeding while waiting for Dr. Grove to arrive.

Two hours later, Dr. Grove looked at his patient who was about to be wheeled into surgery. "You're going to have a few more weeks of recovery without your Jobe shirt." The doctor began to raise his voice. "You ruined all my work! Don't you realize that you run the risk of bleeding out or developing a life-threatening infection? This is not a game. Just because this surgery was not performed as a life-saving procedure, it is still a part of the initial injury and should be treated with the same care. Do you take everything casually if it isn't as bad as the chemical accident? Is that your problem? Do you want to die *after* you've survived the worst?"

Al lay on the table in pain and misery listening and praying for anesthesia. "Sorry."

"Tell your young, beautiful wife you're sorry. She's the one sitting downstairs in the emergency room waiting area worrying about you. I get paid. Do you like coming in for surgery? Call a goddamn repairman next time. Are you kidding me? This is the stupidest, most asinine thing I have ever seen." The angry doctor turned on his heel and entered another room to scrub in for the surgery.

Would somebody give me a break? I'm in pain and he's yelling at me. I know it was stupid but what am I supposed to do, pay someone every time there's something wrong with the house? The sump pump must have shorted out from the overload or maybe it has nowhere to go. What a mess that's gonna be to clean up.

The bed moved and Al felt the temperature change. "Hello, Mr. Plevier. We're going to start the medication into your IV line. Please count backward from one hundred."

Al never got to ninety-five. He was sent home from the hospital later that week and was confined to the living room sofa during the day. The weather had finally broken and some of his friends from construction had come over, cleaned the entire basement, and figured out that the sump pump float had been stuck in the down position. The extension cord for the washing machine had been laying on the basement floor and was the cause of the electric shock he felt.

Banned from wrestling with Albert or handling Larry, Al filled his empty hours by trying to grasp the second level Braille that had become elusive for him. After much effort, he chose instead to utilize level one of Braille combined with a system he invented for his own use and from that point forward never bothered to learn the other levels.

This combination of level one and his own system allowed him to be hired by a local carpet company to make sales calls from his house. As long as he stayed within his area code, he did not have to dial it first. He would start with the number 1 and work consecutively until he had worked through all the numbers. Then he would begin with a new set of the first three numbers in his area code. Although the money was minimal it added to the household, gave him practice with the Braille system, and kept him occupied while he recovered from the electric shock fiasco.

At night, while Elaine watched TV, he occupied his mind by playing logic games as he sat next to her. He would start by the states in alphabetical order and then continue on until Elaine realized he wasn't listening to the program or his mind wandered. Probability problems from college came back to him, and he learned to have the patience to work through them.

If I had taken the time to really think my way through these back in college, I wouldn't have needed help from my buddy, Dan. All the problems I now remember were common sense. He relaxed and thought about his friend. He and Dan both went to the Newark College of Engineering, the only college they could afford. *I remember how disappointed I was that I couldn't afford to go to Texas A&M or Cal Poly. Turned out, I got a good education and it gave me the proximity to see where things with Elaine were going to go.*

"Al, are you asleep or are you working through logic problems? You're quiet." She spoke softly.

He turned his head toward her. "I'm awake, just lost in thought. How can you stand to watch these programs? Listening to it bores me to tears."

She reached over to touch his left hand. "Only another half hour. Thanks for sitting with me."

"No problem. I'll try not to drift off." He returned to the college years that led to his job at A&K.

What if I had gotten into the Air Force like I really wanted? I passed the physical, but couldn't get past the interview with those nine uniformed guys behind the long table. He laughed out loud.

Elaine turned her head slowly. "What's so funny?"

"Sorry. I was lost in my thoughts."

Those professional, older, experienced Air Force interviewers asked me what I thought a chemical engineer did and I mumbled to them that 'a chemical engineer dealt with chemicals.'

"You ready for bed?" Elaine switched off the TV.

"Yes." Al thought a change in subject would bring him into the present. "Do you remember your mom's reaction when

(282)

she first saw this place?" Al laughed.

"Is that what you were so deep in thought about?"

"No, but remember what the yard looked like and the hole in the kitchen ceiling that went through the roof? You could look up and see the sky." Now Al laughed harder. "The house was condemned. The yard looked like the Addams family house. We're lucky we were able to grab it before a builder bought it for the land."

She yawned loudly. "I didn't care what my mom thought. This place was so unique with its stone water well and the river only seventy feet from the house. After growing up in Paterson, I wanted a chance to experience the country."

"You got country. In Paterson, everything was within a block or two, but here if you don't have a car you're screwed." The sound of a baby stirring made them both freeze in place.

"Larry is up to four hours between feedings." The baby's fussing ceased.

"That boy is growing like a weed. I think he's going to be a Linebacker." Al yawned. "What time is it?"

"Around eleven." Elaine snuggled closer to him.

"I'll take the feeding at one if you take the five. I'll get Albert up in the morning, so you and the baby can sleep in." Al relaxed and placed his glasses on the nightstand.

"Are you sure?" She knew Al was feeling better but wasn't sure if enough time had passed for the healing.

"I'll hold him with the left arm." He had learned the hard way to accept his limits.

"Fine. Just don't try to do anything while you're holding him. Put him down first. I don't want to go to the hospital." Elaine rolled over.

Neither do I. "Good night."

Al did let Elaine and Larry sleep late the next morning. She never heard the doorbell at ten. Al ran to answer it, stubbing his toe on a toy in his haste. "Who is it?" He spoke as loudly as he thought he could without waking Elaine and the baby.

From the other side of the door, on the left entrance to the

(283)

house a familiar voice answered him. "Al, how are ya, Buddy? It's Fred."

Al opened the door and stepped aside to indicate that his former construction pal should come in. "Hi, Fred. What are you doing around here?"

Fred reached down and took Albert's hand. "Hello to you, big guy." Albert smiled but continued to hang behind his father's leg. "I'm working across the river on the Michaels house. Al, I don't know how to tell you this, but there is a man across the river taking pictures of your house."

"Are you sure?" The distance across the Pompton Ramapo River was three hundred feet and combined with the property width was far enough away so that he knew Elaine would never see the man from their house.

"The leaves on the trees are gone and that guy isn't trying to hide. He's standing out in the open. Do you know who he is?" Fred stepped all the way inside allowing Al to shut the door.

Busy with the new responsibilities of a second child and Al's recent surgery, he and Elaine had temporarily let the detective have his way with them. This left Mr. Bayplaza to discover the company that hired the detective was BBLvd.

"This started in the fall. He's a private detective hired by one of the companies I'm suing. We haven't heard anything from the neighbors about him hanging around, so I guess he got creative."

The neighborhood the Lake Road house was located in contained about 165 homes with most of the homeowners joining the Pompton/Ramapo River Community. The community members worked night watches, organized picnics and at one point, Al was president of the association. Two highways closed in the small community, creating a triangle that the river served as a backdrop for.

"My lawyer found out BBLVD is paying the private investigator a hundred grand, can you believe that?" Al shook his head and closed the door behind Fred.

Fred made a low blowing noise. "Sounds like a spy novel.

If someone gave me fifty grand I'd take pictures of you."

Al laughed and made a gesture inviting his friend all the way into the house as Elaine stepped from the bedroom hallway carrying Larry. "Hi, Fred. There's someone I'd like you to meet." She held Larry so Fred could get a good look.

The older man looked over the stirring baby. "I think we could use him on the crew in a few years."

"I wouldn't doubt it. Now I need to get him a bottle. You two enjoy your visit. Al, did you feed Albert?" She smiled down at the baby.

"Yes, about two hours ago." The two men walked into the living room and Al sat in the winged back chair to the left of the sofa. "Elaine, Fred saw someone taking pictures across the river."

She shrugged her shoulders under her blue velour sweat jacket. "I'm not surprised. I'll write it down in the log book the lawyer told us to keep." The joy of the new baby distracted her initial reaction of fear.

"How are you doing with the lawyer?" Fred had been to visit Al while he was hospitalized the first time.

"He's good. It's a waiting game." Al turned his head in the direction of the river. "The lawsuit could drag on for years. There's no pot of gold waiting for us."

"There never is." Al's old friend looked admiringly at him. "Plevier, you're one of the most resourceful guys I ever met. We used to call you the scrapper. You'll go twelve rounds with these guys." He joined his tanned and calloused hands behind his head.

"Fred, do you know that if BBLVD can prove I'm fifty-one percent responsible for the accident, I lose?" Al sat up straight in the chair. "And if I win, I have to pay back all the Worker's Comp money I've been getting."

Fred could see his friend growing angrier over something he had no control over and decided it was time for a subject change. "How's the arm?" Fred inclined his head to his friend out of habit.

"Healing, again. I thought the doctor was going to kill me."

"Your wife wanted to kill you." Elaine chimed in from the kitchen where she had started to heat Larry's bottle.

(285)

"It's rude to listen in on private conversations." Al smiled and got up from the chair, still unable to sit for very long without his Jobe shirt. "You want something to drink, Fred?"

"Sure. Soda, if you got it." He watched Al. "You look better than the last time I saw you."

"I was 168 pounds before the accident and now I'm around 185. Must be all her cooking." He crooked his thumb in Elaine's direction.

"I'm happy for you. It looks like you beat this thing." Fred smiled broadly at his friend and then at Elaine.

Al opened the refrigerator to retrieve Fred's soda. "When the hospital calls with a donor cornea available, then I'll feel like I beat it."

Fred's eyes grew wide. "What? That's great!"

"I'm on the list, but first I had to complete the surgery for the chest cavity, and then I have to pass the physical. After that, the waiting begins." Al carried the soda to Fred. "Unfortunately, the reality is that while I'm handed the miracle of a donor cornea, another family faces the grief of having lost a loved one. It's hard to be happy when you think about it in those terms."

Fred, a very religious man, had always wanted Al to join a prayer group. "It would be easy to say the Lord works in mysterious ways, but it would be trite. If it is His will that another individual is called home, we can only pray and be grateful that person respected life enough to consider helping someone else."

Al listened to his friend unconvinced. "I guess, but unfortunately it's my only option. I either agree to go on the donor-recipient waiting list for my temporary reprieve from living without sight, or accept this condition as irreversible." He thought it was worth Fred's time to hear the details of the gift of sight from a donor. "The donor cornea has to be stitched to the remaining rim of the old cornea that goes around the eye and connects to the white. That means scar tissue and the fluid that is supposed to nourish my eye will always be cloudy. Since the fluid will be cloudy, it will make the new cornea cloudy."

Fred held up his hands forgetting Al could not appreciate

the gesture. "You're losing me."

Al stopped and circled back. "The point is that the doctor can't keep doing corneal transplants on my eyes over and over. The more of the scar tissue that is cut, the less remaining cornea there will be to attach it to."

Fred felt the elation leave the room. "I understand."

Al also felt the change. "Fred, I'll take what I can get."

Chapter XXIV: Waiting Game

*F*or Al, the tantalizing prospect of being able to see was overshadowed with the knowledge that someone else would have to die. The corneal transplant was not meant to be a permanent solution for his loss of sight, but could give him the opportunity to see his family for a brief period of time. The time of returned sight was measured by him as eternal. If the surgery was successful, and there had been no permanent damage to the optic nerve during the accident, he would regain sight for about six months.

In April of 1976, Al passed a complete physical conducted by Dr. Westmont and was cleared to be placed on the recipient list for the donor cornea. He was sent to Manhattan Eye and Ear Hospital in New York for the necessary blood work and met with Dr. Leesville who would be performing the corneal transplant. The physical would not need to be repeated unless a cornea was not found within a year of the initial physical. The blood work results, however, were only valid for three months and would need to be repeated accordingly. If he caught the flu or even a bad cold he would have to be passed over for the next person on the list.

Maintaining optimum health that spring became a goal and waiting for the phone to ring became an obsession. In late April, the phone did ring with the possible availability of a donor. Al was told to stay by the phone and wait for a second call to confirm the time to arrive at Manhattan Eye and Ear Hospital. The house came to life as Elaine made the necessary arrangements for a babysitter, and Al gathered items together in a bag to take with him. Eight long hours later, the call came to say that he would be passed over this time for a recipient who was a perfect match.

Al left the bag with a change of clothes and toiletries sitting next to the back door and walked away from the phone. "This is a roller coaster ride. First, I'm pumped up with the possibility of having sight, then I remember the poor person who died, and then the hospital cancels at the last minute. We have to do this over and over. Are you going to be able to handle the stress?"

Elaine tucked her oxford shirt into her jeans. "Are you kidding?" The events of the past year and a half rested between them. "I'll be fine. We knew this from the first time we talked to Dr. Leesville." She picked up her tea mug, now cold from sitting while she prepared for the trip to the hospital. "I'm trying to deal with this as best I can. The hope is more tortuous than exciting."

"I know this is nerve-racking." *I can't wait to hold her close and stare into those blue eyes. I can still see them.*

Elaine looked up from her mug at his fallen face. "We still have hope. The chance for you to have sight is close. We need to learn patience. The doctors never promised us it would be easy or fast or even a definite success."

Al shifted his weight from one foot to another. "I wish we knew one way or the other. I lie in bed and dream about how the two of you looked the day I left for work."

"The chance for you to see the changes in Albert makes the waiting and disappointments bearable." The lines of tension that were visible on Elaine's face seconds before smoothed away.

He continued to shift his weight. "I try not to think that the transplant will be 100 percent successful, in case it isn't." He let his head drop down. "The chemical might have traveled before the emergency room doctor was able to pull it out with the experimental drugs. It could have done irreparable damage to the retina and optic nerve. I may see the difference between light and dark and nothing else."

I remember the look in your eyes when I asked you to marry me and how your blue eyes shone when you said yes. I remember how you smiled and how you cried when I slipped the gold wedding band snugly next to the too small engagement ring. I remember and that is how I can stand waiting to see you, if only for a little while.

"Al?" *He's lost in his own memories. I can't wait for him to see Larry.* "Al? Where are you?"

He brought himself back abruptly. "Elaine, you want to do something tonight? I need to get my mind off the transplant."

"With two kids and a negative budget?" She kicked her shoes off and left them in the kitchen. "Let's order a pizza after the kids are asleep."

Al felt her move to his side and he reached for her hand. "I can guarantee the hospital won't call today, and I need to stop thinking and speculating about what will happen after the surgery. I did have a fraction of light perception, but we won't know anything for sure until the bandages are off. Dr. Leesville would not make me any promises."

Elaine shook her head slowly. "Al, I know all this. Stop replaying the tape for yourself."

He used his free hand to rub at his shoulder under the Jobe shirt. "I still itch a little even with the shirt on. It's always in spots I can't reach." He rubbed at his shoulder, grateful for the ability to wear the Jobe shirt after his fiasco of ripping open the stitches from his surgery. "So, what do you want to do for my birthday?"

"If you want to do the same thing we did last year, I'll have to order more infant formula and diapers." She snuggled close to her husband and placed her head on his left shoulder.

He tried to lift his left arm around her, but the Jobe shirt made it impossible, so he settled for holding her hand. "Let's stay home. I'd rather have a quiet night this year anyway. I don't want to be out somewhere and miss the donor call."

"We can't stay locked in the house. The transplant team said not to do that. The corneas are shipped in low temperatures to ensure preservation. We can get you to Manhattan immediately, if necessary. You can't be a prisoner waiting for your freedom." She adjusted herself further into him. "We made the commitment to try this and now we have to do our part."

"Speaking of doing your part, can you remember to either open doors all the way or shut them?" Al put his left hand to his forehead on the spot he had banged while pacing the house earlier that afternoon.

Elaine looked at the red bump he touched gingerly. "Sorry. Where did you get nailed?"

"Bathroom." He let his hand fall away from the bump.

"I had a few other things on my mind today." Wiggling on the couch she worked her way to the edge of the worn down, too soft cushions. "I'm going to check on the kids. Albert has been sneaking out of bed during naps if he doesn't fall asleep right away." She looked at her husband sitting in his short-sleeved shirt. "You better throw on a sweater or sweatshirt. It's still raining out and the house is damp. You can't risk catching a cold."

"You're right." Al sat on the couch trying to decide what he wanted to do for the rest of the day. He walked to the stereo and felt over and around it for his albums. He touched the pieces of Braille tape located in the top right-hand corner of each album. He found the album he wanted, placed the record on the phonograph, and slipped the headphones on. Music blared and he settled on the floor in front of the stereo in his own private space. This space with blaring music was his comfort zone before the accident. Tonight, under the headphones, he put himself behind the wheel of every car he ever owned, radios blasting.

Man, how many times did I cheat death from behind the wheel of a car?

The record placed him in a summer mood and he thought about the construction job he worked full time at before being hired by A&K. It was the summer of 1972 and he was driving with a seasoned construction veteran, Bill, in Al's used pickup truck. The two men traveled to a job site via Route 23 in the northbound lane. Without warning, the steering mechanism broke on the truck and he found himself crossing into the other lane of oncoming traffic.

The older man grabbed at the dashboard and tried to brace himself for the inevitable crash. "Shit man, do something!"

Al gripped the useless steering wheel, turning it erratically from left to right and hitting the brakes, as the pickup continued to cross over the other lane and toward the opposite shoulder. "I'm trying! I can't do anything!"

Horns blared as a fully loaded dump truck traveling in the southbound lane barreled toward them down the hill. Unable to slam on its brakes and swerve in time to avoid potentially killing other motorists, all the driver could do was head for the pickup. Al was so close, he could see the man's brown eyes.

The pickup finished its uncontrolled veering to the opposite shoulder as Al kept his foot slammed on the brakes. The dump truck roared past the passenger side door within several feet. The pickup truck came to a rest between a tree and a telephone pole in a spray of dirt, grass, and smoke. Al turned off the engine and sat behind the wheel trying to breathe. Wordlessly, the older man fell out of the passenger side door and onto the grassy area where the truck had stopped. Never looking back, he walked the five miles to the construction site in a state of shock.

Al sat behind the broken steering wheel inside the cab of the pickup, stunned. Seemingly out of nowhere, the driver of the dump truck leaned into the already opened window. "Man, what the hell is wrong with you? Steering or brakes go out?" He looked from Al's white face to the open passenger door.

Unable to turn his head yet, Al mutely nodded to the truck driver. A cop pulled up and came running to the side of his pickup.

"Out of the truck!" Believing Al to be drunk, he opened the driver's side door and pulled him to the ground.

The forceful action of the cop brought Al out of shock. "Easy! Something broke with the steering." He felt the officer let

(292)

go of him as his knees gave way and he plopped himself onto the grass. "Can you get a tow truck for us?"

The cop looked at him puzzled. "Who's us?"

Al looked at the cab and didn't see his co-worker. He lifted himself to his knees and then saw the back of his co-worker walking away from them down the highway. The old man never looked back or talked to Al again.

Al put both hands to his head and pulled his knees toward his chest. "Oh, my God! I almost died!"

Remembering that summer day four years ago, Al shook his head slowly as he laid on the area carpet facing a blackened abyss. The album finished playing, but he continued to lie on the worn-down carpet with his arms at his sides, the darkness and silence bringing him quiet respite as Elaine came into the room and sat next to him.

Al lifted off the headphones. "Are both the boys asleep?"

"Deeply. Albert was still clutching his Batman. I had to pry it out of his hands." She snuggled closer and felt the hardwood floor beneath the gold carpet. "Wanna listen to the TV? The couch is more comfortable."

"The floor gives my back a break." He touched her arm.

"You were off in your own little world. You do that a lot now." She stared at him.

He shook his head from side to side. "Sweetheart, I wasn't thinking of anything since the album stopped. Guys just don't sometimes."

"How can anybody not think of anything? Don't you want to talk?" She laid her head back down.

He inclined his head toward the phone and laughed. "I might reconsider if we order that pizza you mentioned."

(293)

Chapter XXV: Celebration

*T*wo more cornea donor alert phone calls and subsequent cancellations caused doubt, but not hopelessness. The young family lived month to month both emotionally and financially. Elaine continued to look for a teaching position, but found no openings within an hour's drive of their home, and Al continued with the telemarketing.

Al and Elaine celebrated their fifth anniversary quietly as the United States was preparing to celebrate its Bicentennial with one of the largest celebrations taking place in Manhattan. Tall clipper ships and the Navy would be in front of the many firework shows in the harbor. The spectacular shows would take place on the East River, Liberty State Park, and other locations around the world's most famous island.

Al's loss of sight diminished the excitement he felt for the holiday and the subsequent firework displays. He did not want to attend the family reunion picnic planned for the fourth of July at the town celebration in Wayne, but never told Elaine. Inwardly he cringed at the thought of sitting in a beach chair listening to the booms and the reactions of the crowd that watched the fireworks. July fourth proved to be humid and hot even for the expected midsummer heat.

He promised himself that he would not let his feelings about the holiday be known to Elaine. "We have to find a spot under the trees." He had put the dishes from breakfast in the sink when the phone rang.

Running his hand along the counter he picked up the receiver. "Hello?"

"May I speak to Mr. Plevier?"

"You've got him." He took a slow swipe across the counter to see if he missed anything.

"I'm calling from Manhattan Eye and Ear Hospital. We have a donor cornea in route and would like you to prepare to leave immediately upon our second confirmation call." The voice on the other end of the line sounded as if she was the same person that had called last Tuesday.

"Thank you. I'll stay by the phone." Al hung up and turned toward the living room. "Elaine?"

She stuck her head out into the living room from the hallway. "Yes? I'm busy getting the boys ready, who was that?"

"It was the hospital. A donor cornea has become available. We need to stay by the phone." *And I'm off the hook for the afternoon in the sun and probably the fireworks.* "I don't want you to miss out on the picnic. It might prove to be another false alarm."

Elaine carried Larry across the living room to where Al stood next to the phone with Albert following close behind. "We can't take that chance. I'll call dad and he can take Albert to the picnic. If we don't hear back from the hospital right away we will stay here with my mom. If we do hear from them, my mom will stay here with Larry if she doesn't want to take him to the picnic. It was going to be challenging bringing a five and a half-month-old to the fireworks anyway."

"Elaine, the celebration and picnic are a big deal. Are you sure you want to miss it?" Al began to shift his weight from one foot to the other as he held out his left hand for the baby to grab.

"Are you kidding? I'll call Mom right now and tell her we're on call." Elaine reached for the phone.

Albert started to climb up his dad and Al reached down and picked up the little boy. "I guess you're going to have to get used to me recovering all over again, little man." Albert squealed with delight as his dad carried him into the living room for playtime.

An hour later when Mr. and Mrs. Hinds arrived, the hospital still had not called the second time. "Where is everybody?"

Albert immediately jumped up away from his toys and ran to his grandfather. "Pop Pop!"

The phone rang as Mrs. Hinds dropped her purse on the counter. She saw Al on the carpet giving Larry a bottle. "Al, I got it." She walked over and picked up the receiver. "Hello?"

"Could I speak to Mr. or Mrs. Plevier?"

"Yes, one second." Mrs. Hinds covered the phone and called Al. "I'm sure it's the hospital. I'll take the baby." She tried to contain her excitement in case it was another false alarm.

Al began to rise with the baby in his arms and felt his right leg had partially fallen asleep. Instinctively he gave Larry a slight hug as he handed him to his mother-in-law, and then walked over to the counter to take the call. "Hello?"

"Mr. Plevier?"

"Yes?"

"This is Manhattan Eye and Ear Hospital. The donor cornea is available and viable for transplant. We have a perfect match for you and need you at the hospital within an hour and a half." The same woman who had phoned earlier spoke quickly this time.

"We'll leave immediately. Thank you for calling. Do we need to call Dr. Leesville?" Al's stomach began to tighten with the anticipation.

"No. The staff will be waiting for you at the emergency room entrance. Good luck to you."

"Thank you." Al's hands shook as he replaced the receiver. "This is it, Mom." Mr. and Mrs. Hinds choked back their tears. "Elaine? Mom is she outside?" He called into the blackness in front of him.

Elaine came out of the master bedroom quickly. "What? Was that the hospital?"

"Yes, this is it. We have to go." Al bent down to hug Albert who had sensed the excitement and run across the room to grab Al's leg. "Albert, Mommy and Daddy have to run out. You stay with Pop Pop and have a good time at the picnic." He lifted Albert and kissed him on the top of the head before calling to Mrs. Hinds. "Dad, we have to get out of here."

"Al, we have everything under control." Mr. Hinds took Albert from Al and the little boy squirmed to get down. "We saw the picnic food on the counter. Albert will probably come with me, but the little guy can stay with your mother-in-law if Elaine stays in The City. Now go."

Elaine kissed the baby on the head and tried to grab Albert for a hug that he quickly escaped from. "Thanks, Mom. Thanks, Dad. I'll try to call from the hospital, but I don't know what we are going to encounter. We've got to try to get into The City in an hour and a half. I don't know if that's going to be possible today. The George Washington Bridge would probably be the best route, but I don't think it will help much. Everyone is going in for the fireworks and boat show."

Al was at the back door holding his small black hospital bag and wondered if the bicentennial celebration would allow them to get close to the hospital at all. "We have to go now."

"Let's go." Elaine was at his side.

Mr. Hinds held Albert high in the air above his own head. "Good luck, Al. Albert, tell Mommy and Daddy bye."

Albert giggled. "Bye, bye, Mommy. Bye, bye, Daddy."

"Be careful driving Sweetheart," Mrs. Hinds called after Elaine as she worried about how her daughter would navigate through the holiday traffic.

Elaine wasn't out of the driveway five minutes before Al also voiced his concerns about her driving. "Honey, I'm worried about you. Getting out of The City is going to be worse than getting in. I don't think you should stay with me. The sooner you get out of The City, the better.

(297)

"Try to relax, Al. I'll be fine. Everyone will be trying to get in when I leave." She gripped the steering wheel tightly as she tried to hide her apprehensions from him. "Let's work toward getting you to the hospital on time. I agree with you about the bridge. The tunnels will have most of the tourists. We can avoid midtown."

Al sat back and listened to the traffic on the highway. It seemed to him that Elaine was passing other cars. *She's really moving.* He thought about the donor and their family. *I hope he or she didn't have small children.*

Al channeled his fears in a different way. "Elaine, I could still be sent home when we get to the hospital. We don't know for sure."

She shook her head adamantly. "I think this is it. You can put all the questions of the conditions of your eyes behind you and move forward one way or another. Today we'll know if you will ever have a chance for returned sight."

The traffic moved without delay as she approached the second half hour of the drive. Within five minutes, the traffic slowed to a crawl.

She stared out the windshield. "What do you think? Should we stop at a phone booth and call the hospital?"

"No." Al was firm. "We'll keep going. There's still parking to consider. I don't think we should stop for anything."

Elaine looked over at Al. Joy and the inevitable fear played across his face and she recited a silent prayer. *God, please give him this reprieve. He needs to catch his breath from all the trauma of the last year and a half.*

The traffic eased and she was able to increase her speed to 45 miles per hour. Al sat next to Elaine lost in his own thoughts. *Elective. How can anyone call this elective? It's a lifeline for me. Even if the operation is a success, it will be like planting a tree in the desert.*

The George Washington Bridge was backed up with a thirty-minute delay, which on this holiday, was to be considered very lucky. Al and Elaine left Wayne at 9:30 am. It was now close to 11:30.   After crossing the bridge, they had to travel downtown to 64th street where the hospital was located.   Elaine wondered if she had made a mistake in not stopping to call and tell the nurses how bad the traffic was.

Al broke into her thoughts.   "Elaine, you can't stay here today while I have the surgery. The nurses and support staff are the best. It's not the day for you to be in The City. I'll be fine." Suddenly Al felt that he would have turned the car around if he thought he could talk her into it.

"We've crossed the GWB. Parking might be impossible. If I can't get within five blocks of the hospital, I'll put on the flashers, walk you into the emergency room, and put you in the care of a nurse. Let's just get there."

Chapter XXVI:
Beginning of the Destination

*A*fter a half hour of circling the hospital, Elaine found an underground garage with one open spot five blocks away. They considered themselves lucky to have found an available garage and exited the car quickly.

"Elaine, I still want you to leave as soon as I'm checked in. It's early enough for you to get out of The City before dark. It's a zoo today." Al had gotten out of the car and opened the rear passenger door to retrieve his cane and bag.

A man leaning behind one of the underground garage pillars finishing the last of a cigarette assessed the vulnerability of a young couple in front of him. The man took one last drag, closed his eyes to absorb his own darkness, stubbed out the cigarette, looked up, and the young couple was gone.

The exit out of the garage was three spaces from their car. Elaine's arm looped lightly through the bend in Al's right arm while he clutched the black bag firmly to his chest. They walked toward the hospital emergency entrance at a quick pace never noticing the man who had raced out of the garage to try and catch up with them or the parking attendant who recognized the mugger's intentions from experience. The normally quiet street was busy with holiday day trippers that either would aid the man's escape or act as would be heroes. The parking attendant stayed close to the mugger and blended into the crowd a few feet behind, until he stopped short when the mugger saw Al and Elaine enlarge the distance between he and them.

Elaine and Al had reached the hospital and rushed through the emergency entrance doors. Standing inside the building Elaine felt like she could catch her breath.

"Let's get you checked in." Positive excitement over Al's admittance to any hospital was a new feeling for her and created a persistent smile in spite of the anxiety she felt whenever he was placed under anesthesia.

Suddenly an older gentleman was at her side. "Excuse me, are you all right?" He was an older man around 70 years old, and he appeared to be out of breath.

"Pardon me?" Elaine looked at the man with a confused expression across her face. "Are you talking to us?"

Al and Elaine had taken their place in the triage line immediately in front of the entrance doors. Already ahead of them was a little girl about eight years old, her eyes covered in bandages, clutching her mother's hand and an elderly woman leaning heavily upon a cane.

The elderly man had caught his breath and continued. "I saw a man following you a couple blocks before the hospital." He inclined his head to Al. "It was an educated guess that you folks were headed here.

Elaine stared at the concerned man as Al jumped into the conversation. "Whoa. What did I miss? "

She shook her head. "I didn't see anyone. Maybe you were mistaken and he was catching a bus."

Al began shifting his weight from left to right foot at a faster pace than Elaine was accustomed to at home. "Al. Try to relax." She let her arm free itself from where it was still looped through his and ran it through her hair. "I didn't see anyone." She turned to the elderly man. "I guess if his intention was to mug us, we outran him."

The short laughter broke the nervous excitement. "I was

coming here also for my wife." The older man paused. "I know what the vulnerability of living without sight creates and I used to work security at one of the big Department Stores in the fifties."

Al cut in with sarcasm. "That's why I'm with her." He moved continuously as he spoke and then stopped suddenly. "How ironic would that be to finally get this close to getting my sight back and then have some punk take it away twenty feet from the front door of the hospital."

The line moved and the little girl and her mother walked to the waiting area. Elaine looked at the older gentleman and wondered how he thought he could have helped. "Thank you for watching out for us. Did the mugger follow us to the hospital?"

The man shook his head. "He slowed down in the crowd. You're safe."

The line moved and the woman in front of them was ushered into the treatment area. Al and Elaine stood before the nurse behind the desk.

"My husband is here for a corneal transplant." The words felt surreal to her.

Al spoke up, unable to contain himself and ignoring the elderly man. "My name is Plevier, Albert Plevier. We would have been here much sooner, but we've been in traffic since nine o'clock this morning. The city is crazy today." His nervous rambling had stopped him from shifting his weight. "Are we too late? Did the cornea go to the next person on the list? We did our best to get here."

The woman behind the desk looked up with kindness. "No, you aren't too late." She pulled a file from the organizer on her desk and looked it over before picking up the phone. "The doctor has not arrived yet, Mr. Plevier. I imagine he is also sitting in traffic. He should be here soon." The individual she was trying to reach finally answered. "This is emergency triage. Mr. Albert Plevier has arrived for a corneal transplant." She hung up the phone and smiled at them. "An Orderly will be right down. I wish you both the best of luck."

Elaine turned back to say goodbye to the older man, but he

had walked away. "Where did he go?"

"What are you talking about?" Al was confused.

Elaine took his arm and move to the waiting area. "The older man is gone. That was strange." A male orderly in his thirties entered the triage area, slowly pushing a wheelchair.

The orderly looked quickly from the little girl with her mother to Al and Elaine and turned the chair toward them. "Hi, folks. Are you Mr. Plevier?" The orderly gave a tired smile as he looked at them for confirmation and received mute nods. "Let's get you upstairs to the fourth floor, so you can rest before the surgery prep. The wheelchair is in front of you to your left."

Al switched his grip on the black bag from his left to right hand and felt the metal arm of the chair. He tried not to jump into it as he guided himself into the leather seat. "Elaine, I think maybe you should get going. I'll be all right. I'm concerned about you going out the same door we walked through. Maybe you could catch a cab back to the garage. The nurses and support staff here are the best."

Elaine held her ground adamantly. "Not yet. I want to stay with you until you go in for the surgery." She followed next to the orderly as he pushed the chair down the hallway to the elevator. "Thank you for being so quick to get us." She looked into the man's face and saw the tired lines around his eyes. "You must be sorry to miss all the celebrations."

The man shook his head and then spoke. "Not really. I'm pulling a double and getting overtime. Working holidays is something you accept in the medical field. We think of it as a normal work schedule." He gave a small yawn. "My wife is used to it."

Al felt the chair turn around as the orderly pulled him back into the elevator. The doors closed and it lifted upward with ease, leaving his stomach with a sensation that made him want to laugh out loud. *I'm so close. This is really happening.* "Thanks for being here today."

The orderly gave a half smile. "You're welcome. You're in the best hands in the business with Dr. Leesville. I'm so happy for you. Most of the patients I work for have lost all possibility of regaining their sight. Their resilience and ability to overcome the heartbreak always makes me appreciate my own life."

Elaine looked at the young man with gratitude as the elevator doors opened onto a floor with patient rooms. "We have every confidence in Dr. Leesville and your support staff. Everyone here has always been wonderful."

Al turned his head toward the conversation. "When you can't see, you are at a complete disadvantage in a hospital, except here. I feel comfortable the minute I walk through the door." He relaxed his grip on the handles of the black bag.

"I'm glad you feel comfortable with us." The orderly indicated his head toward an outside wall and looked at Elaine. "You'll have lots of entertainment with the noise of the cannons and fireworks since we're in the middle of all the shows."

He turned the chair and backed into a private patient room. The room offered space enough for the bed, which extended the width of the room in front of the window, a nightstand and a plastic hospital chair. The hospital was built before the turn of the century, and the size and style of the window reflected this with an accompanying wide ledge. The distance between the bed and the door was about six feet. The room offered a small private bath without a shower just inside the doorway.

The orderly kicked the wheel lock on the chair. "I never introduced myself. Everyone calls me Art." He reached down to take Al's black bag. "Your bed is next to you, on your right, Mr. Plevier. Do you want assistance getting in?"

"No, but it would be great if you could show me where the adjustment controls are." Al stood and eased himself onto the stiff mattress, felt something placed next to him and assumed it was his black bag containing his belongings.

Art handed him the bed controls connected by a thick cord. "Remember, you cannot eat food you may have brought with you. When was the last time you ate?"

"At around 7:30 this morning and I'm starving." Al rubbed

his stomach dramatically.

"Sorry about that, but you're going to be under anesthesia.

A nurse will be in to check your vitals." He looked at the anxious face of the patient's wife. "After Dr. Leesville arrives, a nurse will be in to prep you and move you to the operating room." He pulled the wheelchair backward out of the room saying, "It was a pleasure meeting you both."

"Thanks." Al sat on the bed. "Elaine, I'm settled. You know where my room is and I know where the bathroom is. You should get out of here and out of the city. I'm sure that I won't be waiting too long." He heard her move in front of him. "I need to know you're safe. "Is there a phone in here?"

"I don't see one. When I get home, I'll call the nurses on the floor. I imagine it will take me a couple of hours to get out of the city." She started to give him a light kiss. "I wish I could be here."

"Me too, believe me, but I'll get through this much better if I know you're safe at home." He released her slowly. "I wish I had remembered to pack my radio. Please bring it the next time you come."

Elaine stepped away from the bed. "I want to put the rest of your clothes into your cabinet and walk you through where I placed all of your toiletries in the bathroom."

"I want you to get on the road, please."

"It will only take me a few minutes to arrange your things. You didn't bring much." She opened the closet.

Al hopped off the side of the bed. "Let's get this over with." He walked over to Elaine and felt with his left hand for the bed stand to orient himself. "What are you putting in the cabinet?"

"Your extra underwear and socks will be on the shelf. Your shoes and the bag will be on the floor of the cabinet. There are no drawers." Elaine picked up the bag, moved toward the tiny bath and began to pull out the few toiletries he packed.

He slid behind her in the bathroom and wrapped his arms around her waist. "Are you finished?"

(305)

"Yes. Your toothbrush and paste are on the left side of the sink, your soap, dry shampoo and shaving cream are to the right. The toilet paper is to your left, if you're sitting. Towels, small and large, are on a bar on the wall in front of the toilet, which would be to the right if you're coming in the door." Elaine pulled his arms tighter around her.

"I think I can keep all that in my brain. Now let's get you out of here." He let go of her waist and pulled her left arm slightly to encourage her.

The nurse stepped into the doorway as Al came out of the bathroom. "Hello, Mr. Plevier. I need to take your vitals." The starched white dress the nurse wore brushed the doorway as she entered making a swishing noise.

Al turned in her direction. "Could we have another minute? My wife is leaving and I want to say good-bye."

"Sure." She moved away from the doorway.

"I know I should get going, but I hate to leave you." She allowed him to lead her over to the bed. "I'm not going to the show or picnic today. Larry and I will stay home. I'll call the hospital to check on the success of the surgery later this afternoon. I'll catch the tops of the fireworks from our back yard."

Al sat down on the edge of the bed with Elaine in front of him. He held her waist and tilted his head back. "Be careful. I'm wondering whether that old guy was telling the truth about the mugger."

Elaine laughed. "I think he embellished a little."

"Please take a cab back to the garage. I know it's only five blocks but do it for me. Go out the main entrance instead of the emergency area."

"Al, the way the city is today, I'll be waiting an hour for the cab and then another hour in traffic. I'll be fine, really."

Al felt an uneasy settling in his stomach. "Do it for me or find someone to walk you back to the garage. I don't like this. Don't forget to call and leave a message with the nurses' station. I won't be able to relax until I know you're safe."

She lifted her lips away from his. "I promise."

He let go of her. "Stop stalling."

Elaine watched him and burst out laughing. "I'm going."

"Now, Sweetheart." His serious tone surprised them both.

She turned one more time for her last sight of him looking into nothing. The nurse met Elaine as she left the room. "Drive carefully, Mrs. Plevier." She walked briskly into the room holding the hospital gown meant for Al. "Albert, we're going to check your vitals." The nurse placed the hospital gown on the end of his bed.

"Is there a chance this could be canceled?" Al stammered before he could stop himself.

"As long as you don't have a fever, which would be indicative of your body fighting off an infection, you should be fine." She stuck the thermometer under his tongue and felt his pulse with her right hand. She pulled out the thermometer after a minute and squinted to read the results. "Good, 98.6. Your pulse is strong. Let's check your blood pressure next." She cuffed his left arm and squeezed the pump and announced her opinion. "Everything looks like a go from here. All you need to do now is to wait for Dr. Leesville to arrive and then we will bring you upstairs." The young woman finished writing in the chart and then prepared to leave the room. "I'll be back in a few minutes. Rest. I left the gown at the end of the bed. Please put it on."

Al sat on the edge of the bed trying to gather his thoughts. *I don't know why Elaine or I didn't think to grab my radio. I won't even know what time it is.* He decided to walk the room without his cane so he would have the schematics in his head. He walked around the square which was his universe for the next week and felt for every outlet or anomaly. He climbed back onto the bed and felt the bed control. *I wonder how far these beds can go up and down?* He swung his legs up and laid flat on the stiff mattress. He then pushed the bed into the crunch position as tight as it would go and then stretched it out straight. After raising the height of the bed, he then crunched it. He tried to mix up the controls, started to laugh out loud when he became a little dizzy, and never heard the nurse's shoes as she came into the room to see why the bed was making so much noise.

(307)

"Mr. Plevier, did someone give you the shot to relax you already?" The puzzled middle-aged nurse smiled.

Embarrassed, he quickly lowered the bed and stretched it out. "Nah, I was bored. Do you know how much longer it will be until I'm prepped?"

"As far as we know Dr. Leesville hasn't arrived yet. As soon as he gets here, he will come to see you." She put her hand on the door handle and started to pull it closed behind her as she left. "Try to relax or maybe take a nap."

"Is there still a chance I'll be sent home?" Al vocalized his fear. "I made my wife leave to avoid the holiday traffic nightmare." Al returned the bed to its original starting position.

"There is always a chance something could go wrong, but the donor cornea is upstairs in the operating room cooled and preserved, waiting for transfer. We'll begin to prep you in an hour."

"Thanks. I'd feel like I was in a spa if it wasn't for the slicing I have to go through later tonight. What time is it?" Al adjusted his head.

"Around 3:30. You could be waiting a while." She stood next to the bed. "My name is Sue if you need anything."

"Hi, Sue. How long is a while?" Al turned and rolled to his left side to face the nurse.

"We have no idea. If Dr. Leesville arrives at the hospital and doesn't come up to your room first, we'll let you know he is in the building." Sue walked over to the closet and then came back carrying two blankets that she unfolded and placed over him.

"Ever since I got hurt I'm constantly told to rest or take a nap when people don't know what to do with me. Believe me, living without sight doesn't make you tired, just creative." Al put his arm behind his head and stretched out like a cat. "You do what you have to. I'll entertain myself in here."

The nurse laughed and started to walk out. "The call button is to your left if you need anything. Please change into the hospital gown so you are ready."

"Thank you." Al rolled over.

(308)

She tried to sound stern but couldn't. "Did anyone offer to take your glasses for you?"

"No, but I would prefer to keep them on until I'm being prepped." He reflexively touched the outer rim and adjusted the glasses on his head.

"We want you to be comfortable. I want to make sure your glasses stay with your personal belongings in the room."

The nurse looked her patient over one last time before leaving the room and closed the door behind her.

Al let his mind wander. *I can't believe this. I'm 26 years old and my life has become a fight to exist and my family has been fighting with me.*

He lay on the bed for a few more minutes and then started to play logic games. Solving logic games for him utilized the same principles of engineering that ironically, he could no longer use in a career. Now, when he went to a show or listened to a movie with Elaine, these games kept him awake and sane. These were the lessons of grade school revisiting him in their simplicity and grandeur. These mental games helped him survive mentally and always reminded him that knowledge is not always knowing something but knowing where to find the knowledge. Tapes from the Blind Commission on various subjects including history had been arriving at their house over the last six months. Thoughts of Elaine traveling out of the city brought him back to the present and out of himself.

I hope she is home. It seems like she left a lifetime ago. I hope she listened to me and had someone drive her to the garage. It's no good for her to be walking in the city alone. I need to know she's safe.

Al started to feel himself become tense from worry and decided that he should find a way to divert his thoughts. He began to mentally go over the history tapes he had listened to and tried to remember as many presidents as he could. *I'll start backward, that's the easiest. Ford, Nixon, Johnson...* He then went through the alphabet and tried to see how many words he could make from each letter, then he took groups of letters and made as many words

(309)

as possible.

While Al tried to stay mentally busy, he did not know Elaine had walked out the main entrance of the hospital and toward the garage down a different street, one block over and even busier than the direct route. With one extra block to walk, she quickened her pace, anxious to get home as quickly as possible.

Within fifteen minutes she was in front of the parking garage staring at the attendant's booth. "Excuse me."

"Yes? You're the woman that was with the blind guy, right?" The young man let a newspaper he held drop on the counter in front of him.

"Yes." Elaine felt her body grow cold. "Did you see someone following us earlier?"

"I saw him come out from behind one of the pillars. I swear lady, I never saw him come inside the garage. Not even in a car." The young man worried about a complaint.

"We never saw him following us, but someone else did. Can you please walk me to the car?" Suddenly Elaine felt nervous and a little afraid.

"Sure." The young man quickly walked out of the booth. "He looked like he was surprised to see you moving so fast. I followed him until he gave up. My boss would fire me if he knew I left the booth."

The two found the car and Elaine unlocked the door, wordlessly climbing behind the wheel. She rolled down the window. "Thank you."

The attendant waived to her as she pulled out of the spot and safely started her drive home. Although she left before dark, the challenges of the city rose up to meet her.

Back at the hospital, Al waited for her call. "Mr. Plevier?"

Caught up in his own thoughts, he never heard the door to his room open. "Yes? Who's there?" Al raised himself off the pillows and turned to the voice.

"It's your nurse, Sue." Her soft shoes padded over to the bed. "Dr. Leesville is in the building and will be up as soon as he checks to see that everything is in order."

Al felt butterflies from anticipation. "What time is it? How long have I been waiting?"

"It's 6:30, so you have been alone around three hours."

He dropped his wrist after Sue finished checking his pulse. "Did my wife call the desk?"

"Yes. She said the traffic was horrible in the city. I guess everyone is still coming in for the show." Sue moved around the room preparing something. "She also wanted to let you know she would not be going to the picnic her family is at. Your youngest son Larry will be home with her, but your older son will be going to the fireworks with her parents." Sue laughed. "I think that's the whole message."

"Thank you. I was worried about her." He folded his hands over his chest and felt himself finally relax.

Sue looked at her injured, blind patient and envied the love she knew he and his wife shared. "It's time for you to put on your hospital gown. Don't put it off any longer. I'm not sure how long it will take before the doctor comes up here. There's a lot involved with a transplant, as you can imagine."

"How is the family of the donor doing?" He couldn't help thinking about what this day of a miracle for him meant to the loved ones of the person who died.

"I imagine the family is still in shock. It was a car accident. That is all I can tell you." Sue stood back as Al sat up and swung his legs over the bed. She crossed the room to leave and began to close the door. "Please get changed. If you need help, push the call button."

He felt to his right for the gown and then took off his oxford shirt and then the Jobe shirt. He practically jumped back into the bed and under the thin sheet and blankets. *Man, how low is the air conditioning set in this place? These socks are almost useless.*

A soft knock on the heavy wooden door notified Al that Sue had peeked inside. "How are we doing?"

"I need another blanket. This place is freezing. Why are hospitals so cold?"

"I'll be right back." The young woman retreated quickly

(311)

and returned at a fast pace with another blanket. "See if this helps." She covered him with an additional blanket.

"Are you about five feet five inches tall?"

"Why do you ask?"

"I'm testing myself. I couldn't tell before when I was in the wheelchair. You sound like you had a short stride. How close was I?"

"Not bad. I'm actually five feet six inches and I have long legs. I'd say you're doing pretty good." Another patient's bell sounded and Sue excused herself.

Al listened to the occasional firecracker going off and the continuous sound of city crowds outside his fourth-floor room.

How is anyone getting away with firecrackers in the city?

He listened to the happy mayhem outside and thought about his Albert running wildly around the park at the family picnic.

I'll see him soon, even if it's only temporary. This has to work. I will not stop living on my terms. My boys will have a father who coaches baseball, teaches them to drive, and to swim, and I will show them life is worth fighting for no matter what is thrown at you.

Chapter XXVII: War Zone

While he remained alone in his room waiting for news on his transfer to surgery, Al counted footfalls in the hallway. The tally reached 159 when a set of footfalls stopped outside his door before opening it fully and firmly kicking the stopper down.

It was Dr. Leesville, who entered and stood on the threshold. "Hello, Albert. How are you doing?"

Recognizing the doctor's voice, Al breathed in slowly before speaking, trying to hide his anxiety. "I'm doing fine." Al pushed the button for the bed and rose into an upright position. "Lots of patients tonight even with the big celebration in town?"

Dr. Leesville looked at his patient and saw his tight grip on the bed control button. "Sorry for the delay. Manhattan was a nightmare to drive through. How are you feeling?"

Al turned his head toward the west wall of his room where the sounds from the bicentennial fireworks celebration seemed to tear at the plaster. "I'm a little worried, to be completely honest. How can you operate with all that commotion? It sounds like rockets are just outside my window." He turned his head toward the doctor. "For Pete's sake, don't slip."

Dr. Leesville laughed, but could feel the underlying fear in his patient's voice. "Don't worry. Dr. Westmont and I met at a M.A.S.H. unit in Korea. I'm used to working with bombs going off and constant pressure. This brings back memories for me."

Al tried to relax. "Great."

Dr. Leesville took a long look at his patient. "Time to prepare you for the surgery. I'm going to leave you so I can go upstairs to change and scrub in. The nurses will be in to move you to the pre-op room upstairs." He hoped the tone of his voice conveyed his confidence in the procedure. "I'll see you upstairs, Albert." Dr. Leesville left the room as two nurses came in.

The two new sets of soft footfalls approached the side of Al's bed without an exchange with the doctor. "Mr. Plevier, we're ready for you but first we need to remove your glasses. Where would you like us to put them?"

Al recognized the voice of the middle, aged nurse from earlier. "If you could put them in the closet, I'd appreciate it." The kind woman gently removed his glasses and then turned and placed them on the shelf next to his socks.

Another nurse reached for his left hand. "We have to remove all jewelry."

Al grabbed his hand away and sat on it. "No. Absolutely not. My ring has never been off my finger since the day my wife put it there. It stayed on through the accident, each hospital stay, and emergency procedure. It's not coming off now."

The new nurse was sympathetic and changed her professional tone to one of understanding. "If we don't take it off here, the nurses will remove it before the surgery while you are under anesthesia. If we take it off now, you will know exactly where it is."

"I understand regulations, I've been through the routine, but I will not take off my ring." Al kept his hand tucked.

The nurse shook her head slowly. "I'm going to have to get permission from the head surgical nurse." She padded softly out of the room as the other nurse prepared his first muscle relaxant.

"We need to give you the medication to relax you, but we'll

we'll wait until your wedding band issue is resolved."

After ten minutes the head surgical nurse arrived, stepping no further than the doorway without addressing Al directly. "Jewelry is not allowed in the operating room."

"Then I'm not going." Al's tone was adamant.

All three nurses exchanged looks. "Mr. Plevier, we have a donor cornea upstairs with an entire surgical team ready for your arrival. This has to be resolved now." The head surgical nurse who did not give her name stepped into the room ready to give Al a shot to render him incapable of further debate.

Al felt himself beginning to lose control of the situation and pulled his left hand out from under his butt, to extend both hands and plead his case. "Look, I was burned alive and went through hell during my recovery. Not once did my wedding band come off. It was never even questioned and I refuse to take it off now. I'm able to fight my way back to my life because of this ring." He crossed his hands over his chest.

Silence enveloped the room as the three nurses looked at each other and tried to find a solution. The middle-aged nurse spoke first. "Why don't we wrap gauze around the ring to hide it and then tie the gauze around his wrist?"

The head nurse nodded her head in agreement and then shrugged her shoulders. "You got your way, Mr. Plevier. I think that will work." She nodded at the two other women and began to leave. "By the way, I understand."

Sue returned almost immediately with the gauze. Together two of the nurses wrapped his ring and then prepared the initial medication to relax him. "Ready for your shot?"

"I'm ready, but has this taken too long? Will the cornea dry up?"

The nurse carefully pushed the needle into his right arm. "No, try not to worry. The cornea has been in the operating room and kept cool and sterile." She removed the needle and then moved to the side as two men with a gurney came into the room. "The orderlies are here to take you upstairs."

One of the orderlies surveyed the room. "We're going to

have to remove the nightstand."

The two men wheeled the gurney back into the hallway and came in to move the small night table outside the door. Al then heard the gurney come back in and be pulled lengthwise next to his bed. All the movement seemed to be happening so quickly that he wasn't sure if it was the medication that made him perceive it that way or his nerves. His stomach tightened, but he pushed back the covers anyway and prepared to climb onto the gurney as the cool air smacked into him.

"Would you bring my blankets? It's cold as winter in here."

The orderly tried to help guide him during the transfer, but quickly realized Al needed no assistance. "Sure. We'll strip the blankets off the bed."

Al found his place on the gurney and felt the blankets laid over him. "Thanks." He pulled them up to his neck as the gurney rolled into the hallway. The temperature dropped a few more degrees and Al felt it immediately. *I might as well have paper over me.*

Al was amazed at how the noise from the celebration in Manhattan was able to penetrate the walls of the hospital. Although muffled, the noise had grown louder in the last half hour with the crowds enjoying the spectacular fireworks displays. For Al, it felt and sounded as if he were in the middle of the crowds. The doors to the elevator closed and then opened upstairs on the operating floor. The muffled noise did not lessen. The excitement of the celebration was everywhere and growing.

The gurney entered the OR Prep room and a nurse changed places with the attendants. She began gently inserting an IV into Al's left arm. "Hi, Mr. Plevier. How are you doing?"

He listened to the escalating joy outside the hospital walls and knew in his heart that he would soon have a chance of joining a crowd. "I'm ready. Knock me out."

She patted his arm for reassurance. "You're still in the OR Prep, but I am about to wheel you inside the operating room where you'll receive sedation. Dr. Leesville has scrubbed. You two will meet in the operating room before you are completely asleep."

Al felt the gurney move and the air changed. It was sterile and even cooler than the air in the prep room. He still heard the bicentennial celebration except that it was now more muffled and consisted of continuous booms without the crowd noise. He felt the gurney nudge into a solid object.

"Mr. Plevier, we need to move you one more time onto the operating table." A nurse on his left and one by his head were ready to guide him. "Please put your right hip over to the table first. Don't worry the wheels on the gurney are locked." Al felt the covers pulled off of him as he slid his hips onto the table followed by his legs. The nurse at his head held the IV bottle and gently moved his left arm to a table that extended to his left where the gurney had been. He heard her hang the IV bottle on a pole above his shoulder.

Al felt the presence of another person next to his left shoulder. "Hello, Mr. Plevier. I'm Dr. Michaels and I'll be your anesthesiologist."

"Do a good job," Al dead panned.

The good, natured man laughed softly. "I promise."

"Hello Albert. Ready?" Dr. Leesville stood behind Al's head, his sterile-gloved hands held up and his face hidden behind a surgical mask. "We're going to give you the anesthesia before we begin to drape your face. I'll see you in recovery."

Al took a long deep breath.

Dr. Michaels moved to his permanent position on Al's left and began to push the contents of the needle into the IV line. "Albert, I'm injecting you with the anesthesia. It will sting a bit. Please start to count backward from one hundred."

"3,2,1. It's not working."

Al heard a collective soft laugh and then the muffled booms of celebration outside grew more frequent and formed a cacophony that rattled air inside the sterile environment and lulled him into oblivion.

Chapter XXVIII: Battle Won

*T*wenty-one and a half months locked in the dark and overcoming tremendous obstacles of pain management, only served to strengthen Al's spirit as he gradually joined the world of the sighted during his recovery. He approached week two following the corneal transplant to the right eye as any engineer would, watching the progress and observing improvements. Al held no fantasy in his mind of one emotional moment when the bandages were removed and he could see crystal clear. The doctor had already explained to him that he would see a gradual improvement if the surgery was successful. Each day in the hospital, as the doctor lifted the bandages to irrigate, observe and medicate the eye, Al first saw an increase in brightness followed by a differentiation in the shadowing of figures. Now he was seeing brief and gradual increased glimpses of his environment with color.

As he prepared to leave Manhattan Eye and Ear Hospital, he gauged his progress with excitement. "Doctor, I can see green and blue today on your shirt collar." Al smiled as he lay back while the plastic shield and then the bandages were replaced over his eyes after the doctor's daily exam.

(318)

Dr. Leesville smiled broadly as he stood back to observe his patient. "Very good. Your progress is where it should be. You'll see gradual improvement this week at home each time you administer the drops to your eye." The doctor turned and spoke quietly to the nurse.

"While I'm still here is there anything I need to know?" It was still frustrating to Al that people with sight sometimes treated him as if he were invisible.

"Sorry Albert. As you heard, we were making notes in the progress chart." The doctor turned his complete attention back to Al. "We can assure you now, that the initial attempts immediately after the accident to pull the chemical out of your eyes with the experimental drugs, were worth the risk. It reduced the damage to the right eye and will enable you to have vision. The limit to the amount of damage was evident during the surgery. The proof will be evident as you begin to see."

Al spread his hands in a gesture of the obvious. "Absolutely. Even if it's temporary, I don't care. I'll always be grateful for the quick thinking of Dr. Westmont that went beyond saving my life."

Dr. Leesville nodded his head. "Ready to go home?"

Al lay on the bed in his street clothes with one foot over the other. "Doctor, I have a six-month-old at home that I have never seen."

Elaine came into the room and casually walked to Al's bedside. "How are you, Sweetheart?"

"Ready. We have a follow-up appointment in three days to see when the bandages can come off." Al sat up straight. "Dr. Leesville said I'm doing great."

Elaine smiled at the doctor and took hold of Al's hand. "We're ready to take care of him at home."

The nurse standing next to the doctor spoke for the first time. "His paperwork is signed. As soon as the chair arrives you can go." She looked toward Al. "We'll miss you around here, but we're happy for you."

The orderly with a wheelchair arrived. Al and Elaine said

their respective goodbyes to everyone. It struck Al how the second most important departure from a hospital was carried out with the same tempered enthusiasm as the drive from Overlook two years earlier. The drive home and his arrival were both uneventful. He found himself three hours later sitting on the living room couch with a sleeping Larry in his arms and Albert playing at his feet.

"Albert, Daddy will be able to play catch with you in a week or two."

Albert climbed onto the couch next to Al. "Daddy, trucks."

"We'll play with those after your mom takes the baby, but won't it be fun to play catch?" Al knew he could learn to toss the ball to Albert without sight, but he wanted the dream he always had since Albert was born.

"Daddy trucks." Albert began rolling the truck across to Larry.

Al felt something move over the baby and he reached out as Larry was about to kick. "Let this little guy sleep." Albert rolled the truck over his brother again and Larry woke with a wale. *Great.* Al lifted the baby to his shoulder trying to soothe him back to sleep and then finally gave up. "Elaine?"

"What is it?" Elaine took one look at the still wailing baby and Albert trying to run his trucks over Al. "Here, I'll take Larry. You play with Albert."

Al relaxed the rest of the afternoon and into the evening with his family. He found himself unable to leave Albert and showered him with attention. Elaine applied drops to Al's healing eye according to the schedule sent home from the hospital and later that night listened to him describe more improvement in his vision as he sat at the breakfast bar.

"Elaine, I can see the outline of the furniture. The color differentiation is not sharp, but I can tell deeper colors from each other." Al swallowed hard. "I can see where the furniture is." Al had a hard time finding his voice. "I can see Albert. He looks like a shadow, but I see the outline of his body by the sofa."

Elaine felt her throat constrict. "Amazing." She was tempted to let Al continue to look around. "Let's cover the eye up.

I'm not taking any chances with infections. We're going to follow the doctor's orders precisely." She covered Al's eye with the plastic cap and bandages.

"This is a miracle of modern medicine." Al held his hands on Elaine's hips as she finished with his bandages.

"We are the fortunate few. I can't wait for you to see Larry and Albert." She moved away and tucked all the medical paraphernalia into a bag and then put it on top of the refrigerator.

"When is my office visit with Dr. Leesville?"

Elaine came back into the bedroom. "Thursday, but he said you won't be completely healed until next week."

"I know. Believe me, I do not want to screw this up." Visions of the chest surgery and his debacle stood out in his mind.

The couple spent the next three days in the routine of administering Al's drops three times a day. Each time he would tell Elaine to what degree he was regaining his vision.

The first time he saw the blurred image of his wife he almost cried. "You still have blond hair."

Elaine looked at him with tears in her own eyes. "Did you think I would change it?"

"I can't wait to see you clearly." He hugged her tight.

At the office visit, Dr. Leesville confirmed that by the end of that week Al should be able to remove the bandages permanently. This seemingly miraculous moment was with the understanding that he would need to continue the eye drop medication and to prepare for the eventual return to darkness.

Al looked up at the blurred image of the doctor. "Doctor, I understand any sight I gain is temporary. Since the day I woke up in the hospital and you told me the operation was successful, I have been steeling myself for the day it fades. The darkness closing in will hurt like hell, but at least I have this. I don't want to spend the next my time with sight talking about preparing myself to live without it. I'll be preparing myself every day as the sight diminishes." Al watched the blurred images disappear as the doctor replaced the protective cover and bandages over his eye.

The doctor stepped away and began to write in Al's file.

"After what I have seen in this exam, I believe the healing is so perfect, that by the end of this week, you may see clearly. You will obviously be the first person to tell us."

And he was. Seven days later Al sat on the edge of the bed and unwrapped the bandages for himself. He lifted the protective plastic cover, prepared to administer the necessary drops, and opened his closed eye to a world that had cleared even further. The previous night the distinction between objects was the clearest it had been since the surgery. In the living room, the color of his red sofa pronounced. Now this morning as he sat on the bed, the blurriness was gone. His vision was not perfect, but he could now see.

He placed the drops in his eye, finished, and reached for the glasses that had one dark lens and one clear lens. The protective glasses wrapped themselves tightly around his head, almost as the goggles had done, to protect the recent surgical work. Carefully Al walked out of the bedroom to look for Elaine. It was the first time he attempted to walk with his new vision.

I thought this would be easy and I'd run to her but, I feel like I'm going to trip over my own feet. I can't stop looking down.

Without thinking he reached for the cane he saw hanging from the bedroom door handle.

What am I doing?

The natural light beamed through the windows to welcome the new day. Looking at his feet, Al made his way down the hallway and prepared to walk across the living room with sight for the first time in almost two years.

Albert looked up from his spot at the breakfast counter where he sat in his booster seat. "Daddy."

"Hi there, Albert." Al noticed that Albert's hair was dark just as it had been the last time he saw him in the same place, but this time in a 'big boy' chair. *Aristotle was right: "While everything changes, everything remains the same."*

Elaine stood up from the lower cabinet in the kitchen and looked at her husband across the room. "Al, can you see me?"

(322)

Al stared at Elaine from the top of her head to the tip of her feet. "You look better than ever." Carefully he walked toward his family, never breaking his gaze as he looked from Elaine to the boys. "Larry." Al reached down and picked up his second son from where he sat in his playpen.

Larry tilted his head back the second he felt Al lean over the side. Meeting his father's stare, he smiled widely and reached for the protective glasses covering Al's eyes, gurgling with delight at his father's image.

Elaine lifted Albert out of his chair and walked over to join them. The four stood together before Elaine could find her voice. "How do we look?"

The clear, crisp, images of his smiling wife and children were framed by the morning sunshine streaming through the window behind them, on a morning similar, but different, to one a lifetime ago.

Al paused, savoring the timeless moment. "Beautiful."

End Book I

Thank you for reading "Beyond the Eight-Foot World" Book I of the Albert Plevier Trilogy.

Please follow the continuation of Albert's story in Book II of the Albert Plevier Trilogy: "See Saw".

Book III: "Changing Tides" is expected to be released in 2019.

For information on speaking engagements with the author and Mr. Plevier, please contact the author:
jaynemkellyauthor@gmail.com

Follow us on Facebook at
www.facebook/thealbertpleviertrilogy.com

Beyond the Eight Foot World

48277265R00185

Made in the USA
Columbia, SC
11 January 2019